Heal With Essential Oils

Joy Burnett

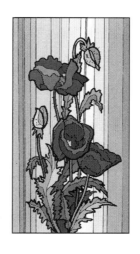

Copyright © 2018 Joy Burnett

ISBN:9781720172192

This book is available as an e-book and in print
from Amazon

CONTENTS

INTRODUCTION

The essential oils of flowers, herbs, trees and shrubs are true treasures. This book is aimed to bring you the wisdom of them in a salient and accessible way.

We've come full circle in medicine and are returning to understanding the incredible potency of plants. A body of knowledge has been accumulated over the millennia through observation, use, and the skill of thousands of practitioners.
Every home should have an essential oil first-aid kit, a natural way to care for many different health problems, especially if it helps to avoid pharmaceuticals, most of which have harmful side effects, pollute our waterways and environment, and are often the reason that our hospitals are so full.

This book is crafted to be your go-to resource for all things related to using essential oils safely and effectively. It will empower you to approach the primary common health concerns affecting most people today.

In it there are ideas and recipes of essential oil blends that promote hormone balance, help reduce inflammation, improve digestion, increase immunity, reduce pain and so much more.

The contents of this book are for informational purposes only and are not intended to be a substitute for professional medical advice, diagnosis, or treatment. Always seek the advice of your physician or other qualified health provider with any questions you may have regarding a medical condition.

NATURE HAS THE ANSWERS

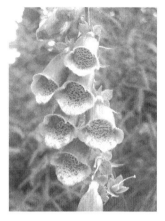

When you start to understand the power of plant extracts a whole world of possibilities is waiting for you. Extracted from flowers, herbs, trees and grasses **Essential Oils** are concentrated, complicated cocktails. They are the odorific principal of the plants, not really oils at all but complicated mixtures of many different *chemicals* such as *esters, terpenes, oxides, phenols, lactones,* and *aldehydes.* They are usually secreted from *glands, ducts,* or *cells* in one or several parts of the plants.

It takes 10lbs of **Jasmine** blossoms to produce 5 mls of essential oil and at least 60 roses to produce a single drop of **Rose** oil. It becomes obvious why those oils are so expensive.

The strength at which any essential oil is used is very important. **Study the chapters on Uses, Applications and Proportions.**

Essential oils are complex in their molecular structure and very powerful. **Digitalis,** which is the essential oil of foxglove, is highly poisonous in large concentrates, but used carefully in medicine, it relieves heart conditions. **Oregano** oil is 26 times stronger as an antiseptic than phenol – which is the active ingredient in many commercial cleaning materials and some of the antifungal oils (**Thyme, Lemongrass, Tea Tree** etc.) are more effective than most pharmaceutical fungicides.

Oils should not feel greasy, and although the consistency and colours of essential oil vary, they should feel fluid and non-oily.

Every essential oil is antiseptic to some degree. Some are analgesic and some renowned for encouraging a sense of well-being. Essential oils are distinguished in many ways. Read the chapter on how they are described. By doing so you will soon learn what they can be used for. For instance, oil that is described as a **Febrifuge** is known to be able to reduce a fever.

Even those well versed in essential oils will benefit from this thorough approach. With your new-found knowledge, you will be equipped to begin tailoring your use of essential oils to meet your unique health needs and lifestyle right away – and start experiencing amazing results!

The healing power of plants is often displayed by the plant itself and according to medical historians studying the activity, shape, colour or other quality, the plant indicates which part or function of the body it will treat. A good example is the **Aloe Vera** plant, which is renowned for healing wounds. When cut the plant will release a drop of gel but will rapidly and visibly draw together the two edges of the leaf and seal the cut.

Paracelsus (1493-1541) wrote, 'Nature marks each growth according to its curative benefits'. **Dioscorides** (40-90

AD,) a Greek physician and pharmacologist, who worked in Ancient Rome, also believed in the **'Doctrine of Signatures'**. He developed a painkiller from the extract of willow. It is from this substance that our most famous analgesic has been derived, Aspirin. It is recorded that the Egyptians, Sumerians and the Chinese also used willow bark as a traditional analgesic.

Nicholas Culpeper who wrote the most famous 'Complete Herbal' in 1653 was an adherent of 'The Doctrine of Signatures'. He was the first herbalist to write directly for ordinary people so that they could use plants in their daily life for health and well-being. Even **Hippocrates**, the 'Father of Medicine', who was born in about 400 BC, extolled the benefits of plants to ward off disease.

Early man lived in a world full of dangers and it is believed that they had natural and highly developed instincts that contributed to their survival. Their sensory perceptions were much more finely tuned to nature than ours are now. Through their senses of observation and smell, it was soon discovered that certain berries, leaves and flowers made sick people better, or their juices healed wounds, or that burning certain woods would induce a feeling of calm for those who breathed in the fumes. Also, they learned simply by observing how animals instinctively used medicinal plants when they were ill.

Burning aromatic plants in religious ceremonies is still used today in the form of incense, **Frankincense** being the most commonly used in churches. This has the ability to deepen breathing, which calms the mind, thus creating a state inducive to prayer and meditation.

In France, fumigation with aromatics to prevent the spread of infectious disease remained in practice until relatively recently. Juniper, Rosemary and Thyme were used because of their antiseptic and antibacterial properties.

What we know as modern "aromatherapy" was not introduced formally until French chemist **Rene Maurice Gattefosse** first coined the phrase in 1937. Although he wasn't necessarily a natural health advocate, he became interested in essential oils after a 1910 accident, where he badly burned his hand. He used the first available salve in his laboratory: a pure, undiluted lavender oil compound, that not only immediately eased the pain, but healed his injury without infection or scar.

Because of Gattefosse's work, **Dr Jean Valnet** used the best essential oils to treat injured soldiers in the second world war, and this led to **Marguerite Maury** being the first person to 'individually prescribe' an essential oil in a healing combination, using a Tibetan technique for back massage, that treated nerve endings along the spine.

Since then, essential oils for healing have become a staple in massage, and alternative and complimentary medicine across the world.
The complex network of molecules in essential oils can deliver strong effects on the body. Their power to beat disease is so effective that, you may be able to avoid having to use needless drugs or have unnecessary surgeries. If you are unsure, find a natural health practitioner or a clinically qualified aromatherapist to give you guidance.

Research now suggests that most, if not all, disease begins with inflammation.

Natural anti-inflammatory properties are critical to the health of the entire body, and are shown to play a crucial role in supporting cardiovascular, neurological, gastrointestinal, immune, joint and connective tissue systems.

Essential oils are known harmonisers: this means they are balancing and trigger homeostasis (the ability to maintain and heal) in the human body.

You'll soon be armed with over 50 recipes for every health need, and a special section for women's health includes dozens of formulations for PMS, fertility, pregnancy, candida, and menopause. Another section on skin problems and how to use essential oils on children.

10 MUST-HAVE OILS FOR YOUR HEALTH CARE KIT

There is a great deal of information available about essential oils, their aromas and uses and for the best in terms of health issues. I have narrowed the list down to the top 10 starter essential oils that combine well, and can be used for many different complaints. These oils have not necessarily been chosen for their aroma alone, but with the idea that good combinations can treat and help many disorders.

These are my suggestions: **Clove – Eucalyptus – Ginger – Lavender – Lemon – Oregano – Peppermint – Rosemary – Tea Tree – Ylang Ylang.**

With these ten oils you can make dozens of combinations.

Examples:

An uplifting blend would be **Lavender, Rosemary** and **Lemon**.
A relaxing blend would be **Lavender, Ginger** and **Ylang Ylang**.
For high blood pressure a mix of **Lemon, Lavender** and **Ylang Ylang**
For a severe cold **Eucalyptus, Ginger** and **Peppermint**.
To use when studying **Rosemary, Clove** and **Lemon**.
For bronchitis **Clove, Lemon** and **Rosemary**.

For pain relief **Oregano, Ginger** and **Lavender.**

For immune support **Tea Tree, Peppermint** and **Lavender.**

SEE RECIPES FOR DETAILS OF INDIVIDUAL COMPLAINTS

Experiment. Find out what suits you and start small.

Read carefully the chapters on **PROPORTIONS & USES, and INDIVIDUAL RECIPES**

BUYING ESSENTIAL OILS

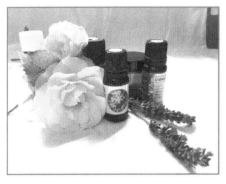

Firstly they must be organic and of the very best quality. Unfortunately, we can get no absolute guarantee of purity. The reality is that it's becoming increasingly difficult to find truly pure, clean air, food and water mainly because of modern agricultural methods and pollution on a massive global scale. This is especially true for supplements and essential oils that are labelled organic.

When buying essential oils, make sure that they have the Latin name on the label so that you can identify the different chemo-types.

For example: **Rosemary** – Rosemarinus officianalis c. borneol/cineole/verbone. This will help you understand their uses.

Although there are many synthetic copies of essential oils and products that are mixed ready for massage, it is only the pure natural oil that is therapeutic and effective on a health level.

Knowing where to buy them isn't as simple as it may seem. My advice would be not to settle for anything but the best you can afford. Find a company that you can put your faith in. They will usually be happy to provide you with information. With trial and error you will find oils that you respond well to. You could contact someone you know who uses essential oils. Most Aromatherapists have a favourite supplier.

Try a couple at a time, and test for yourself. **Lavender, Lemon** and **Peppermint** are relatively inexpensive and you should get a good gauge to see if the brand is for you or not.

Some essential oils can have medication, medical condition, or even age-related contraindications. Check with the appropriate resources to determine if particular essential oils are suited for your health status before implementing the recommendations in this book.

If you are not sure if something is appropriate for you, we suggest working with a qualified aromatherapist to help determine your personal needs.

Each essential oil has biochemical individuality and getting to know their qualities helps you build customised blends for different issues. Using them regularly is one of the most beneficial and economic ways to improve your health and reduce environmental toxins in your home by using fewer expensive commercial products.

Once you have started your collection, it is important to understand that they evaporate, discolour and go off if not stored properly. They must be bought and kept in dark glass bottles to maintain their effectiveness, as it has been shown that plastic-type containers leech into the essential oils (as they do into most things). This will produce hormone disruptors that will contaminate the oil.

Most oils will keep for a long time. The citrus oils do not keep as well as others, and should be used within a year of purchase. Some like frankincense can last indefinitely. Keep your oils in a dark cupboard or box.

The cosmetic and cleaning product industry does use plastic. In these products it is likely that the essential oils used are either synthetic or poor quality.

I encourage everyone to look at Robert Tisserand's website to get more concise information about the subject.

The volatility rate of most essences fall into one of the following three classifications:

TOP NOTES – The smallest molecules and the fastest acting, the quickest to evaporate, the most stimulating and uplifting to mind and body. They contain mostly highly volatile, small molecules and the aroma will therefore last only about 24 hours.

MIDDLE NOTES – Mixed sized molecules, moderately volatile, primarily affect the functions of the body. They are balancing oils and contain a mixture of high and low volatile molecules. They will last 2 to 4 days.

BASE NOTES – Heavier molecules, slower to evaporate. Sedative and relaxing. It is worth noting that a mixture of top note with base note will hold back the volatility of the top note. Being mostly low volatile molecules the aroma can last up to 6 days.

You can check the volatility of your oils by putting a drop on paper and smelling at regular intervals. You will soon see that the top note lasts the least amount of time.

When you have successfully used and experimented with your first ten, add the following to your fragrant pharmacy: **Geranium, Cedarwood, Frankincense, Hyssop, Ravensara and Clary Sage.** With this range of oils you can treat almost anything. They will protect your general health by stimulating the body's own natural healing mechanisms. Also keep your house fragrant, clean, germ and bacteria free.

Next to include in your collection are the citrus oils, **Orange, Lemon, Mandarin, Grapefruit** and some more of the spice oils, **Aniseed, Cinnamon** and **Turmeric** that can be used not only for health but also for cooking as well as cleaning.

Read In The Kitchen on Page 84.

USES and APPLICATIONS

Because they are so potent, they must be diluted in one way or another. They do not combine well with water, so either mix with a basic unscented cream or lotion, milk, honey or base oil like almond, coconut, or grape-seed. Properly diluted, most oils are safe.

There are several methods of use for Essential Oils:

Through the skin: the skin is a sponge and everything you put on it should be free from unnatural or artificial chemicals. Permeability varies throughout the body. Our skin is also our largest organ of elimination. It only takes about 20 minutes to completely absorb most of the tiny molecules that make up essential oils. After approximately 90 minutes they are naturally excreted. They will not accumulate in the body because of their 'high mobility'.

Applied to the skin, whether in massage or application to specific areas, the oils enter the blood stream by diffusion (the volatile oils turn to a gas in liquid form and enter the body via the sweat and oil glands and hair follicles). Large amounts of subcutaneous fat will impede absorption and elimination, as will water retention and poor circulation. Not all the molecules will be absorbed into the body, as some will evaporate.

An aromatherapy massage is one of the loveliest forms of healing. It can be relaxing, restoring, nurturing or stimulated, according to the oils used. The benefits of massage are usually cumulative and can be used as a preventative medicine as well as a curative one. A good practitioner will mix you an 'individual prescription'.

In a bath: Add up to 10 drops of your selected oil mixed with ½ cup coconut milk or base oil and ½ cup of salt. This makes a fantastic soak for circulatory, muscular, respiratory, skin and sleep problems. Choose your oils carefully.

Generally, it is advisable to avoid potent oils that could irritate the skin such as **Cinnamon, Oregano** or **Clove;** instead, use the soothing oil **Lavender, Orange, Geranium, Chamomile, Mandarin, Eucalyptus Radiata** or **Ylang Ylang.**

Foot bath: Lovely for tired, aching feet, fungal or skin problems (See recipes). Also a suitable treatment for those who are immobile, infirm or post operative. Put 3 to 5 drops into a bowl of warm water and soak for 10 to15 minutes.

As a compress: 10 drops in 1 tbsp. proof alcohol added to 4 oz. of water. Soak cloth and apply for bruises, infections, aches and pains. (See recipes) Wrap in cling film.

For swelling and inflammation cool a cloth in the freezer before use.

Where heat is needed use hot water.

Inhalation: Essential oils enter the blood stream by the interchange of gases in the lungs. The lungs are lined with a rich blood supply, which readily absorbs the essential oil molecules. These then travel around the body before they are eliminated. The tiny molecules also enter directly into the nervous system via the **Olfactory Nerve**.

The Olfactory centre is very closely linked with the *limbic system* in the brain, the seat of our emotions and feelings. This extremely active system is connected to other vital parts of the brain involved in controlling heart rate, blood pressure, breathing, memory, and reaction to stress.

Certain oils stimulate specific neuro-chemicals within the nervous system. Therefore smells can evoke pleasant or unpleasant responses and memories, can affect the mood and general well being. As every single person is different, it is important to use oils that you are familiar with and like.

For quick inhalation, use a bowl of hot water and add 2 to 4 drops of your chosen oil. Drape a towel over your head and the bowl. Inhale for a few minutes.
Another way is to add 2 to 4 drops of your chosen oil to water and put into a vaporiser, or add to a professional steamer.

Direct inhalation should not be used by asthmatics.

Anosmia is the complete lack of the sense of smell but according to Essential Oil Safety Expert **Robert Tisserand**. He states 'As far as we know, psychological effects do not take place for someone who has completely lost their sense of smell, but the physiological effects still do.'

What we know about the olfactory system is still limited. However, you should still use essential oils regardless of whether you can smell them or not.

Ingestion of essential oils is controversial. Like many other things, they are poisonous and if administered in the wrong way or with the wrong dosage they can create serious irritation to mucus membrane. However, the food industry uses about 50% of the essential oils grown for flavouring and they flavour almost everything we eat. Many liqueurs, yoghurts, jams and fruit drinks are flavoured with rose oil. Sausages and meat products are flavoured with spice and herbal oils. The citrus oils are not only in many foods but also in cleaning and medical products. Within the food industry there are strict guidelines for the use of oils in food and because they are mixed with food substances they are easily ingested.

There are two reasons that it is not a good idea to put essential oils in water to ingest. One is that essential oils do not dissolve in water, so it makes it more difficult for your body to assimilate the oil into its system. And secondly, taking them this way would mean that the tiny molecules are floating around in your stomach, which could lead to irritation of the very sensitive mucus membrane lining of the intestines.

One could argue that because essential oils are produced naturally by plants and we have been ingesting plants without any problems for centuries it should be quite safe to take them internally. But, within plants, essential oils are found in naturally balanced mixtures and the individual oils molecule are 'quenched' by the other ingredients.

I have personally taken essential oil internally many

times. Just 1 drop of **Clary Sage** in a teaspoon of almond oil for a nasty period pain. For a serious bronchial infection, a combination of **Eucalyptus, Oregano** and **Rosemary** in almond oil and in a soft gel veggie capsule. In food, I have added one drop **Turmeric**, one drop of **Marjoram** and 1 drop of **Oregano** to a lamb stew. And once on holiday, I took in water (no carrier oil available) 1 drop **Tea Tree** and 1 drop **Peppermint** to ward off a virulent tummy bug that was attacking everyone in the hotel where I was staying. It worked!

My conclusion is that taking essential oils internally may be a very effective method to get the oils to be absorbed into the body to help extreme problems. Very small doses are recommended. Never exceed recommended dosage.

Creams and Lotions: For general body care, add 50 drops of essential oil to 200 mls base lotion. **For facial creams see recipes.**

Salves: A 2% dilution is recommended, which is 12 drops per 1 ounce of oil.

SAFETY and PRECAUTIONS

Are you sure that you are using essential oils safely and effectively? Are you confused by dilutions and conversions? Let's make sure you know how to dilute your oils. As explained in the previous chapter, not all oils are safe, so it is wise to understand all the individual precautions and contraindications before embarking on using them.

If we are to use essential oils safely in our own homes, it is necessary to be aware of the problems that can arise from their misuse. They will serve you well if you observe a few basic rules.

- Never use undiluted oils directly on the skin. One or two of the oils can be used neat in certain circumstances but do not be tempted unless you know exactly what you are doing.

- Dilute your oils with cream, carrier oil, lotion, alcohol, milk or flower water depending on what you are going to use them for.

- Avoid contact with eyes. Wash with carrier oil if an essential oil gets into the eyes, and consult a doctor if the irritation persists.

- Avoid exposing skin treated with oils to sunlight, especially the citrus oils, **Lemon, Bergamot, Orange, Grapefruit** and **Mandarin**. These are phototoxic but are only really a risk if applied in high doses.

- Certain oils should not be used if homeopathic remedies are being taken, particularly **Eucalyptus**, **Oregano, Camphor, Hyssop, Basil** and **Peppermint**, which can neutralise the effect of the remedy.

- Essential oils that are not stored well do go off and can cause an irritation or an allergic reaction. They are not the same thing but they look similar. If you have an irritation reaction once you stop using the product and remove the oil from the skin, then the reaction dies down very quickly. With an allergic reaction, it tends to remain inflamed for many hours, sometimes longer than that, and it will come back every time you use the same product in the same dilution. Basically if you have an allergic reaction then your immune system has created antibodies to something in the product or the blend you have used, and you can assume that you will have that allergic reaction for life. So you really want to avoid them.

- Always store your oils in a cupboard in dark glass bottles.

- Ingestion of essential oils is not recommended unless a full qualification in Aromatology is achieved or under the supervision of a qualified Aromatherapist. (**See previous chapter**)

- Observe the rules that apply to age, gender, general health and during pregnancy. **Read section on Pregnancy.**

- Do not use cheap or adulterated oils.

- Stick to recommended doses.

- Oils are highly inflammable so keep away from naked flames or excess heat.

- The following oils are considered unsafe for home use: **Bitter Almond – Baldoleaf – Calamus – Yellow Camphor – Horseradish – Mugwort – Mustard – Pennyroyal – Rue – Sassafras – Tansy – Thuja – Wormseed – Wormwood.**

- Half doses are generally used for children and the elderly. **Read chapter Essential oils for children.**

- **ALWAYS ENSURE THAT THEY ARE OUT OF THE REACH OF PETS, CHILDREN,** and the **INFIRM.**

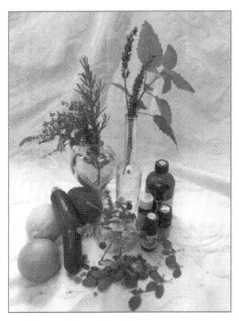

Preventing sickness has to be proactive. A body that has been ravaged by tobacco, junk food, alcohol, anxiety and stress or overwork and neglect will not respond overnight to any kind of natural remedy. But, it is never too late to improve your health. True healing takes time and it has to be combined with a change in **nutrition, life style and attitude.**

Using essential oils can help many disorders, but for the best results it should form part of a **Holistic Health Regime.**

Whatever your usual routine first thing in the morning it should start by drinking a large glass of warm water. You can add a slice of **Lemon** (cleansing), a teaspoon of **Turmeric Powder** (anti-inflammatory), a teaspoon of **Manuka Honey** (loads of health benefits), or some grated **Ginger** (gut cleansing and anti-cancer.)

Breathe deeply for about 30 seconds. Anyone can do that, even if you have a heavy, rushed schedule. Open your throat and pull the breath into your body filling the stomach, then the rib cage and finally the upper lobes of your chest. Those breaths can be combined with a conscious effort to relax your body and use a positive affirmation:

'Today <u>is</u> a beautiful and special day.'

'Today, everything I *do* is successful.'

Not *might be*, or *perhaps*. It *will* be special. Bring it into the Here and Now. Create a positive day before you start it. There is a saying, 'FAKE IT TO MAKE IT'. So start to create your own health, success and happiness.

It is impossible to avoid environmental toxins and synthetic chemicals. As much as we possibly can we should be trying to minimise them. The air that we breathe affects our health and even the health of a baby in the womb. Therefore it makes sense to reduce as much as possible the use of artificial chemicals in the home and garden.

We need to look for the underlying causes of the presenting symptoms and treat the whole body. The oils will stimulate rather than suppress the body's natural defence mechanisms.

It seems foolish to use the NHS for trivial, minor complaints that can be dealt with easily with essential oils. About 80% of patients use antibiotics unnecessarily.

We must value our doctors to treat serious disorders, but we should not take it for granted that they should treat everyday sniffles, headaches, aches and pains or skin problems.

Natural therapies generally speaking do not relieve instantly, which is what we have come to expect from our medicines. They are not magic potions but they assist the healing process, which happens automatically in the body with the right fuel, treatment and conditions.

The chemistry of each of us is different and even as we age we change. What suits us at twenty-years-old does not necessarily suit us at fifty.

Trillions of micro-organisms live on and in the skin. It is highly absorbent which means that we can easily absorb toxins through it. All those commercial products we love to use can be full of untested chemicals that are used to create them and they are absorbed directly into our blood stream.

Read the labels on things like shower gels, body lotions, sun tan creams and face creams. So many have unnecessary and harmful ingredients. Some toxins found in sundry beauty and cleaning products include phenoxyethanol, parabens, and formaldehyde.

It is relatively easy to make good skin and body creams that contain no harmful chemicals by using natural products and adding essential oils. They can have highly beneficial results. A few recipes are included in the skin care section.

Using essential oils can have quite a dramatic effect on the body. Those suffering with sinusitis, cramps, PMT, and migraine, insomniacs and arthritics have found these problems have been helped with a sustained use of essential oils. Over a of three to four weeks is the best way to judge the effects.

OIL DESCRIPTIONS

This list is by no means exhaustive.

ANALGESIC   Relieves pain
ANTIFUNGAL   Prevents and treats fungal infection
ANAPHRODISIAC   Decreasing sexual desire
ANTICONVULSIVE   Prevents convulsions
ANTIDEPRESSANT   Alleviates depression
ANTIDIABETIC   Improves circulatory problems
ANTI-INFLAMMATORY   Reduces inflammation
ANTISEPTIC   Inhibits the growth of bacteria
ANTISPASMODIC   Relieves spasm especially in smooth
                         muscle
ANTISUDORIFIC   Reduces perspiration
ANTIVIRAL   Inhibits viral infection
APHRODISIAC   Increases sexual desire
BACTERICIDAL   Inhibits and treats bacterial infection
BECHIC   Reduces or relieves coughing
CARMINATIVE   Eases colic and flatulence
CEPHALIC   Mental stimulants for poor concentration
CHOLAGOGIC   Stimulates the flow of bile to the intestines
CICATRISANT   Promoting healing and the formation of
                         scar tissue
CORDIAL   A tonic for the heart
CYTOPHYLACTIC   Stimulating the production of new
                         cells
DECONGESTANT   Helps diminish catarrhal blockage

DEPURATIVE	Blood cleansing
DETOXIFYING	Helps cleanse body of impurities
DIURETIC	Stimulates the secretion of urine
EMMANOGOGIC	Hormonal balancing
EXPECTORANT	Helps removal of phlegm and catarrh
FEBRIFUGE	Helps reduce fever
GALACTOGOGIC	Increases secretion of breast milk
HAEMOSTATIC	Stops bleeding
HEPATIC	A tonic for the liver
HYPERTENSIVE	Raises blood pressure
HYPOTENSIVE	Lowers blood pressure
INSECTICIDE	Insect repellent
IMMUNOSTIMULANT	Supports the immune system
NERVINE	A nerve tonic
PARTURIENT	Aids childbirth
RUBERFACIENT	Warming. Stimulates circulation locally
SEDATIVE	Calming. Inducing sleep
STIMULANT	Increasing activity and wakefulness
STOMACHIC	Tonifies the stomach
TONIC	Invigorating
UTERINE	Giving tone to the uterus
VASODILATOR	Causes small blood vessels to expand
VASDOCONSTRICTOR	Causes constriction of the blood vessels
VERMIFUGE	Eliminates intestinal worms
VULNERARY	Helps healing of wounds

HOW ESSENTIAL OILS ARE DESCRIBED is really important to know. For instance oil that is described as **Antispasmodic** can be utilised to give support both energetically and physically. Physically, they are used to help relieve muscle spasms and cramps of both voluntary and involuntary muscles. Physical issues that would be considered spasmodic could include menstrual cramps, tight muscles after a work out, an asthma attack, or a spasmodic cough. Many of the oils in this category tend to be especially effective when used to support the particular organ or system that the oil has an affinity for. For example, **Rose oil** could be specifically indicated for the reproductive system (think menstrual cramps) while **Peppermint** would be better suited to supporting the respiratory system. When choosing which oils to use for spasmodic conditions, take a few extra minutes to study the different oils you're considering. Getting to know your oils over time will give you the tools you need to choose which will be most effective for the particular situation.

Oils with antispasmodic properties can also be useful when dealing with emotions. Use any of the following oils to help release feelings of pressure, anger, frustration, fear tightness, tension, anxiety or feeling cramped. **Chamomile, Frankincense, Patchouli, Neroli, Ylang Ylang** and **Lavender.**

PROPORTIONS

Proportions are important and the following is a guideline only:

If essential oils are being used as preventative measures (Immune support, circulation, etc.) extended or regular treatments are recommended. If the treatment is for symptomatic relief, short-term use is enough. Treatments for chronic conditions such as rheumatoid arthritis, M.S, diabetes, lung disorders or permanent digestive issues may need on-going and regular use and treatments.

Preparing Massage Oil or Lotion for the Body

A general guideline for the amount of **carrier oil** is dress size for ladies (size 12 = 12mls) or chest measurement halved for men (40ins halved 20ins = 20mls)

Typical Massage Strengths:

12 mls carrier oil.	Maximum 6 drops essential oil.
20mls carrier oil.	Maximum 10 drops essential oil.

Initially use only three oils to make your blend. Learning to use your nose as an indicator is just as important as getting the right mix. It may be made up of drops from 2 to 4 different essential oils.

When using a mixture of essential oils it is a good idea to put them together in one bottle or jar. With this method you can then make massage oils or lotions easily and economically and also have some oil left over for a bath, for inhaling, or to use in the next bottle of carrier oil or lotion.

To 50 mls of carrier oil or lotion: 15 to 25 drops of essential oils.

To 100 mls of carrier oil or lotion: add 30 to 50 drops of essential oil.

To 200 mls of carrier oil or lotion: add 60 to 100 drops of essential oil.

10 ml cream 1 to 2 drops essential oil.

DOSES SHOULD BE HALVED FOR THE ELDERLY AND YOUNG CHILDREN.

CEDARWOOD – CEDRUS ATLANTICA

Distilled from the wood of the tree. It is a yellow to deep amber, viscous oil with an aroma that is warm and woody with a hint of balsam and turpentine. Native to the Atlas Mountains of Algeria the oil is mainly produced in Morocco.
There are other species of Cedarwood and the oldest recorded is Cedrus Libani from Lebanon, this was most probably the oil used by the Ancient Egyptians for embalming, building and shipbuilding.

PROPERTIES: Antiseptic, Antibacterial, Aphrodisiac, Antispasmodic, Astringent, Diuretic, Expectorant, Fungicide, Insecticide, Sedative, and Tonic.

USES: The warm, woody scent of Cedarwood produce a grounding aroma that promotes feelings of vitality and wellness. Mixed with Rose or Lavender it has a sedative effect and is good for anxiety and tension. It helps to calm the mind. When you find yourself distressed by unfamiliar situations, inhale the aroma of Cedarwood oil to promote calming emotions. Put it in a diffuser at the end of a long day when you want to create a relaxing environment. Use three to four drops with three or four others of your choice. (Patchouli, Lavender, Orange).

Before exercising, massage one to two drops onto your chest (suitably diluted) to maintain vitality throughout your workout. It helps respiration.

Its astringent qualities make it ideal for acne, fungal infections, greasy skin, dandruff, and hair loss.

Cold and chest infections respond well to this oil. It has the ability to break down mucus, so it helps with the treatment of catarrhal conditions, especially chronic bronchitis.

It is a useful oil for problems of the genito-urinary system and particularly helpful with cystitis. It has a tonic and cleansing effect on the kidneys and lymph.

Good for general aches and pains.

Considered to be a sexual stimulant, it is used extensively in masculine perfumes and after-shave.

Cedarwood oil provides a simple solution for repelling insects in the home. Place a drop of Cedar oil on a cotton ball and place in closets, storage boxes, or other areas to keep moths at bay. When the aroma fades, replace the old cotton ball with a fresh one or add another drop to ensure that no bugs will make their home in your furniture or storage areas.

BASE NOTE WHICH BLENDS WELL WITH: Rose, Lavender, Juniper, Patchouli, and Benzoin.

CAUTIONS: Do not use Cedarwood produced in the U.S.A. They are a different species and have different properties. These oils are used mainly in the perfume industries and are not suitable for therapeutic purposes. Cedarwood is a good substitute for the more expensive Sandalwood.

CHAMOMILE GERMAN – MATRICARIA CHAMOMILIA

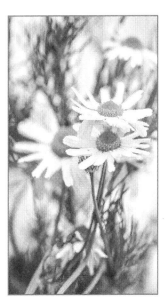

Steam distilled from the flowers of the plant, the oil varies from pastel blue/green to dark greenish/blue. The oil from Matricaria Chamomilia is usually very dark in colour because of its high Azulene content. Azulene is a powerful anti-inflammatory agent that is not actually present in the plant but is formed in the production of the oil. Therefore Matricaria Chamomilia is a more potent remedy for inflammatory conditions than other chamomiles like Anthemis Nobilis, known as Roman Chamomile. Matricaria has a refreshing earthy aroma and was at one time cultivated in Germany, hence its name. There is another Chamomile available; *Ormenis Mixta or Moroccan Chamomile,* which possesses similar properties to the true chamomile but it belongs to a different botanical family.

PROPERTIES: Antispasmodic, Antiseptic, Antibiotic, Antidepressant, Anti-inflammatory, Antineuralgic, Anti-phlogistic, Carminative, Cholagogic, Sedative.

USES: Invaluable for skin conditions such as eczema, urticaria and dry/flaky conditions. As skin problems are often related to stress responses, Chamomile is invaluable as both a sedative and anti-inflammatory treatment. Use in cold compresses for swellings. It has been used successfully on burns, inflamed ulcers, and boils. As it is carminative it soothes the stomach, relieving gastritis, diarrhoea, colitis, nausea and may be helpful when treating irritable bowel syndrome.

Good for female disorders, including scanty menstruation, painful or irregular periods, and excessive loss of blood during long periods and menopausal problems. Its action on the liver makes it useful for treating jaundice. On a psychological level

Chamomile is good for anger and heated emotions. It is often useful to use when insomnia is due to anxiety, over excitement or excessive worry. Being so gentle it can safely be used on children and the elderly.

It is best blended with other oils as it has a strong aroma on it's own. Roman Chamomile is less pungent.

MIDDLE NOTE WHICH BLENDS WELL WITH:
Benzoin, Bergamot, Geranium, Lavender, Lemon, Neroli, Rose, Patchouli and Ylang Ylang.

CAUTIONS: Should be avoided during the early months of pregnancy. There have been a few rare cases of people who have developed dermatitis following the use of this oil.

CINNAMON — CINNAMOMUM ZEYLANICUM

Steam distilled from the bark, twigs and leaves. The chemical content varies but both are equally useful. Cinnamon-leaf oil is less expensive than the bark oil, mainly because the leaves are more easily harvested than the inner bark. Most of the usage and flavour of cinnamon comes via its bark, which has less eugenol, (a phenol which is a highly antiseptic and anaesthetic chemical). The lingering warmth of the uniquely sweet aroma of cinnamon is matchless.

PROPERTIES: Anaesthetic, Antimicrobial, Antispasmodic, Analgesic, Antibacterial, Antidepressant, Antidiabetic, Antifungal, Astringent, Antiseptic, Cardiac, Carminative, Detoxifying, Emmenagogic, Haemostatic, Immuno-stimulant, Insecticide, Galactagogue, Stomachic, Vermifuge.

USES: As a spice it is one of the must-have's in your kitchen rack.

Unsurprisingly, cinnamon has been prized for centuries as part of traditional Ayurvedic medicine. Because of its phenol content it is often used in Indian and Arabic meat dishes. This chemical will destroy bacteria and prevent putrification. It is found in the spice mix garam masala.

Because of its properties it is useful against infections like colds, and flu. Used in a burner it will help prevent infection spreading.

Applied locally it will help relieve the pain of diarrhoea,

menstrual cramps, constipation, aches and pains, digestive disorders, circulatory problems and general sluggishness.

Because of its benefits to the circulation, it is a good oil to use for diabetics in a massage. Taken in food (the powder rather than the oil) it helps lower blood sugar levels.

It has a calming and a sweet aroma that instantly soothes your mind and the soul. Inhaling cinnamon essential oil can help boost brain activity and improve blood circulation.

Last, but certainly not least, is cinnamon ability to fight cancer. Eighty studies to date have investigated cinnamaldehyde's capacity to inhibit tumour cell proliferation via trigger cancer cell apoptosis (programmed cell death) and other mechanisms and the research is clear: cancer patients should be encouraged that natural solutions truly do exist!

BASE NOTE WHICH BLENDS WELL WITH: Lavender, Ylang Ylang, Rose, Rosemary, and all the citrus oils.

CAUTIONS: Aldehyde and Eugenol are known skin sensitizer and should be used with great care. Highly diluted and combined with the gentler oils it can be applied for local areas and body massage. Even as a potentially sensitizing and irritating oil, we shouldn't make the mistake of avoiding cinnamon altogether.

CLARY SAGE - SALVIA SCLAREA

Steam distilled from the flowering tops of the plant, plus leaves and stalks. The oil is clear to pale yellow green, and it has a warm, sweet nutty odour. The best oils are produced in France and Hungary. Sometimes called 'eyebright' because water distilled from the leaves and flowers can be used to bathe the eyes to clear away soreness and give them a sparkle. *Sclarea* – Latin for clear.

PROPERTIES: Antidepressant, Antiseptic, Antispasmodic, Anticonvulsant, Aphrodisiac, Astringent, Carminative, Deodorant, Emmenagogic, Hypotensive, Nervine, Parturient, Sedative, Stomachic, and Tonic.

USES: It is strongly antispasmodic so it is useful in any condition that needs calming such as pre-menstrual cramps, inflamed skin conditions, or digestive problems. It helps relieve asthma as it relaxes the bronchial tubes. It is a powerful muscle relaxant so it is especially useful where muscular tension arises from mental or emotional states.

Used in the last stage of labour to improve the efficiency of uterine contractions. During childbirth, Clary Sage oil and chamomile oil are the most effective in alleviating pain.

It can induce dramatic and colourful dreams so take care not to use it with alcohol as nightmares might result. It is renowned for its ability to produce mildly euphoric states and is therefore considered to be an aphrodisiac.

Because of its ability to control heat in the body it can be used by menopausal woman and by people fighting disease and to combat the night sweats experienced.

It reduces blood pressure and helps with mood swings and PMS, muscular and joint pain.

Clary Sage is known to affect the hormones of the body because it contains natural phytoestrogens, which are referred to as 'dietary oestrogens' that are derived from plants and not within the endocrine system. These phytoestrogens give Clary Sage the ability to regulates oestrogen levels and ensures the long-term health of the uterus – reducing the chances of uterine and ovarian cancer.

A lot of health issues today, like infertility, polycystic ovary syndrome and oestrogen-based cancers, are caused by excess oestrogen in the body – in part because of our consumption of high-oestrogen foods. Because Clary Sage helps balance out those oestrogen levels, it's an incredibly effective essential oil.

TOP NOTE WHICH BLENDS WELL WITH: Ginger, Geranium, Juniper, Neroli, Marjoram, Lavender, Cinnamon, Sandalwood and the Citrus oils.

CAUTIONS: Can be very sedative. It is best used in a persons own home so as they will not have to drive after their treatment. It affects concentration and can often have an effect on the practitioner. Generally, safe oil due to its high content of esters and alcohols. Not to be used in the first 6 months of pregnancy.

CLOVE - EUGENIA CARYOPHYLLATA

This oil is extracted from the buds, the unripe fruit and the leaves. All have similar chemical constituents. However the oil from the bud is usually of superior quality. It is sweeter, richer, and warmer.

PROPERTIES: Analgesic, Anaesthetic, Antibacterial, Antifungal, Antiseptic, Aphrodisiac, Antispasmodic, Carminative, Cicatrisant, Insecticide, Parturient, Stimulant, Stomachic, and Vermifuge.

USES:
Clove oil acts as a general tonic for both intellectual and physical weakness. It is said to be helpful for frigidity, impotence and sexual problems (diffuser only). As its odour intensity is high, it is a great mental stimulant (use for tiredness when studying) effective against respiratory problems (use in a diffuser).

It is beneficial in treating inflammatory conditions such as rheumatoid arthritis and other musculo-skeletal conditions. It adds a rich, warm aroma in a massage treatment. For a full body massage (1 drop only) blended with Orange, Lavender and Black Pepper it is also a wonderful immune stimulant.

It has a high proportion of eugenol (a highly antiseptic and anaesthetic chemical) is commonly used for oral infections and to kill a wide spectrum of microbes including staphylococcus aureus and pseudomonas aeruginosa, two

41

bacteria that often lead to pneumonia and skin infections. Also controls E. coli.

Put it into a diffuser to relieve nausea.

This oil is used extensively in the food, cosmetic, and the perfume industries.

BASE NOTE WHICH BLENDS WELL WITH: Lavender, Orange, Grapefruit, Cinnamon, Black Pepper and Basil.

CAUTIONS: It should only be used in the minutest dosage. It is very potent and can cause skin irritation.

EUCALYPTUS - GLOBULUS / RADIATA / SMITHII

Steam distilled from the leaves and young twigs of the tree and it produces a pale to dark yellow oil with a strong distinctive antiseptic aroma. Radiata and Smithii are both gentler than the Globulus and can be used by the whole family. There is also available as an essential oil, Eucalyptus Citradora, which has a distinctive lemon tang. It is used extensively in the cosmetic and perfumery trades. It has many of the properties of the other eucalyptus varieties and is extremely safe and is lovely for massage mixed with Geranium, Ylang Ylang or Lavender.

The majority of Eucalyptus oils are now produced in Spain, Portugal and Brazil.

PROPERTIES: Analgesic, Anti-catarrhal, Antibacterial, Anaesthetic, Antifungal, Antispasmodic, Antirheumatic, Antimicrobial, Antiseptic, Antiviral, Aphrodisiac Astringent, Cicatrisant, Decongestant, Expectorant, Febrifuge, Insecticide, Rubifacient, Stimulant, and Vermifuge.

USES: Like clove essential oil, eucalyptus essential oil has a profound effect over staphylococcus infections. Quite amazingly, recent research showed that when staphylococcus aureus comes into contact with eucalyptus oil, the deadly bacteria completely loses viability within 15 minutes of interaction.

This highly antiseptic oil is so useful for any infections of the respiratory tract such as colds, flu, laryngitis, bronchitis, sore throats, croup, sinusitis, and rhinitis.

Radiata is effective when treating upper respiratory tract infections i.e. Mucus conditions, catarrh, sinus and head colds. Direct inhalation is recommended.

Used in a burner or diffuser, it will purify the air to stop infection spreading.

Eucalyptus is also excellent in blends for muscular aches, neuralgia, rheumatism, and joint pains. Its action has a pronounced cooling effect on the body.

Helpful with malaria, measles, diabetes, cystitis, ulcers, sores, burns, blisters, lymph node infections, headaches and neuralgia.

The Aborigines have used this oil for treating almost every malady for centuries.

It is also used extensively in the pharmaceutical industry, in flavourings and toiletries.

TOP NOTE WHICH BLENDS WELL WITH: Lavender, Geranium, Rose, Neroli and Marjoram.

CAUTIONS: Often rectified. Better not used on highly sensitive people or children. Eucalyptus Radiata or Smithii are gentler. Not to be used with homeopathic remedies.

FRANKINCENSE – BOSWELLIA CARTERII OR THURIFERA

Also known as Olibanum it is distilled from the resin from a small tree from China, the Middle East, Ethiopia, Lebanon, and North East Africa. The gum resin does not occur naturally in the tree but is produced as a protection when the bark is cut and it produces a milky juice, which hardens. It has a clear, refreshing odour, slightly spicy and the oil is a light golden colour. It improves with age.

PROPERTIES: Analgesic, Antiseptic, Astringent, Carminative, Cicatrisant, Cytophylactic, Digestive, Diuretic, Expectorant, Immuno-stimulant, Sedative, Tonic, Uterine and Vulnerary.

USES: This oil is best known for its ability to deepen and slow the breath and it has a calming effect on the mind and body. Throughout history it has been used traditionally in the form of incense for religious ceremonies. It produces a state conducive to concentration and meditation.

It is a useful oil to use during a counselling session or at any time when it is necessary to produce a relaxed and trusting atmosphere. It is considered to be a 'mind' oil, as its action on the nervous system produces a feeling of calm. It's comforting action is helpful for anxious or obsessional states linked to the past. Because of its beneficial effects on breathing, it is useful for treating asthma, laryngitis, bronchitis, and coughs.

Frankincense essential oil has also been used with much success to treat issues related to digestion, the immune system, oral health, respiratory problems and anxiety.

It is invaluable for the treatment of cystitis and urinary infections. It is found to be effective on wounds, sores, abscesses, ulcers, acne, and inflammation and particularly for its cicatrisant properties for scarred skin. Its astringent properties help balance oily skin conditions. Said to be an effective treatment for nose bleeds.

In Ancient Egypt it was used for fumigation, preservation and perfuming. In Africa it was used to keep insects at bay.

BASE NOTE WHICH BLENDS WELL WITH: Geranium. Lavender, Ylang Ylang, Cinnamon, Black Pepper, Patchouli and the citrus oils.

CAUTION: Although a very safe oil it is not considered suitable for use on children.

GERANIUM – PELARGONIUM GRAVEOLENS OR P. ADORATISSIMUM

Steam distilled from the leaves and shoots. The oil is a pale green in colour and has an aroma with the sweetness of Rose and the sharpness of Bergamot. A great deal of this oil is used in the perfume and cosmetic trade. Most varieties originate from South Africa and there are several hundred different species. The best oils come from Reunion; others come from France, Italy, Corsica, Spain and North Africa.

PROPERTIES: Analgesic, Antiseptic, Antidepressant, Antidiabetic, Astringent, Cicatrisant, Diuretic, Haemostatic, (anti coagulant principle in leaves), Insecticide, Sedative, Tonic, Vulnerary.

USES: Circulatory and lymphatic, so it is excellent for treating cellulitis and any sort of congestion in the body. Helps diabetics and because it is good for circulation it helps with any condition where there is inflammation or infection.

It helps kidney functioning so therefore it can help with water retention.

It is one of the oils that help hormone regulation so it is useful for problems such as PMT, endometriosis, infertility, and menopause. It particularly helps with breast problems such as engorgement or mastitis

In skin care it is invaluable as it can be used on any skin type and it is especially helpful for acne and eczema. As it assists healing it is good for skin problems and can be used for minor wounds, rashes, burns, ringworm and shingles, herpes simplex and athletes foot and it helps alleviate dandruff.

It is often effective in mouth and throat infections, where it acts as an analgesic.

It alleviates depression and anxiety and it stimulates the adrenal cortex.

MIDDLE NOTE WHICH BLENDS WELL WITH:
Most other essences but especially with the citrus oils.

CAUTION: Often falsified with cheaper oils. Very occasionally causes dermatitis.

GINGER – ZINGIBER OFFICINALE

Extracted from the root by steam distillation, the oil varies from very pale to deep yellow. It has a pungent, warm, spicy aroma and is not really what one expects.

PROPERTIES: Analgesic, Antiseptic, Anti-spasmodic, Aperitif, Aphrodisiac, Bactericidal, Carminative, Cephalic, Expectorant, Febrifuge, Laxative, Rubifacient, Stimulant, Stomachic, Tonic.

USES: This highly important spice has been used since ancient times and its medicinal and culinary uses are widely recognised throughout the world.

For the digestive system it is renowned for being a stimulant to the whole system. It is excellent for flatulence, colic and nausea and helps with travel and morning sickness. Mental fatigue and motion sickness don't stand a chance with Ginger in hand.

It is used in traditional Chinese medicine for many purposes but particularly where the body is not efficiently coping with moisture.

A few drops added to a foot bath can be very helpful when suffering from colds or flu. For sore throats it is affective as a gargle. It's rubifacient qualities make it invaluable for the treatment of arthritis, cramps, stiffness, fibrositis, poor circulation, and water retention.

It is purported to have Aphrodisiac properties and has

been used successfully through the ages to help flagging sexual appetites.

The Romans used it for eye infections and diseases.

In the Middle Ages it was used to counteract the black death. It promotes sweating.

It is used extensively in the food and perfume industries.

BASE NOTE WHICH BLENDS WELL WITH: Most oils.

CAUTIONS: Not suitable for highly sensitive skins and it should never be used neat.

HYSSOP – HYSSOPUS OFFICINALIS

Hyssop has a long history as a cleansing herb. It is mentioned in the Old Testament in that context. It is used for flavouring Benedictine and Chartreuse liqueurs. Although it should be used with caution, it does have some valuable therapeutic uses, as can be seen from the following list of properties.

PROPERTIES: Antiseptic, Antispasmodic, Astringent, Bactericidal, Bechic, Cardiac, Carminative, Cephalic, Cicatrisant, Digestive, Diuretic, Emmanogogic, Expectorant, Febrifuge, Hypertensive, Nervine, Sedative, Stimulant, Stomachic, Sudorific, Tonic, Vermifuge, Vulnerary.

USES: This is excellent oil for respiratory complaints: coughs, colds, bronchitis, influenza. It reduces mucus and bronchial secretions and spasms.

Hyssop oil neutralises the Tuberculosis bacillus at 0.2 parts per thousand.

Relieves gout, arthritis, rheumatism and tension pain.

It is useful used in a rub for the abdomen for constipation, wind, and menstrual pain.

Although considered good skin oil as it has a healing effect, it is most useful for bruising and scars.

In many ways it is stimulating oil and it can create alertness and clarity, cleansing emotional grief and pent up feelings.

Hyssop montana/canescens, which is a different

chemical construct to officinalis, is considered one of the best oils to use for asthmatics (not directly inhaled as this can worsen the effect).

CAUTIONS: Do not use during pregnancy, or if you suffer from high blood pressure or epilepsy and do not use in a diffuser near anyone who is pregnant or has these conditions. Do not use on the elderly or children.

LAVENDER – LAVENDULA ANGUSTIFOLIA OR LAVENDULA OFFICINALIS

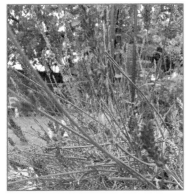 Steam distilled from the flowers, leaves and shoots. The oil is colourless to pale yellow with a sweet, floral-herbaceous aroma. Indigenous to the Mediterranean, it is now cultivated all over the world.

There are many different species of Lavender – stoeches, spike, hidcote, dwarf blues and bowles are just a few.

PROPERTIES: Analgesic, Anticonvulsive, Antidepressant, Anti-inflammatory, Antiseptic, Antispasmodic, Carminative, Chologogic, Cicatrisant, Cordial, Cytophylactic, Diuretic, Emmenagogue, Haemostatic, Hypertensive, Hypotensive, Insecticide, Nervine, Rubifacient, Sedative, Stimulant, Sudorific, Tonic, Vermifuge, Vulnerary.

USES: Generally regarded as the most versatile essence therapeutically and can be used for almost every conceivable complaint.

It is especially known for its power to help attain deep restful sleep.

Reams have been written about Lavender oil and it is regarded as the most useful oil to have as it can add a pleasant aroma to some of the less pleasant smelling oils.

It is non-toxic and non-irritant. It is one of the few oils that can be used directly onto the skin.

Well-known for its calming properties, lavender is wonderful for accelerating healing of burns, cuts, stings, and other wounds. It is jam-packed with antioxidant power. Scientists have discovered that lavender essential oil helps induce a decrease in oxidative stress, which is known to cause heart disease and many other health concerns, as well as increase antioxidant enzyme activities.

Certainly it is worth using this oil in the treatment of diabetes and heart disease. As it is both hypotensive and hypertensive it is invaluable for controlling blood pressure.

Lavender is probably the most adaptable oil available as it can exert a cooling or a warming effect on the body depending on the dosage and what is being treated. Conditions such as fever, congestion and inflammation a low dosage (less than one per cent) is recommended. This will have a cooling, calming effect whereas with cold, chills and fatigue, a higher dosage will generate a warming reaction.

MIDDLE NOTE WHICH BLENDS WELL WITH: All other oils.

CAUTIONS: One of the least toxic oils but care should still be taken as the cheaper Lavendin is often sold as Lavender.

LEMON – CITRUS LIMON

Pressed from the rind of lemon, the oil is a pale yellow and has a sharp tangy refreshing smell. The best oils come from India, China, Japan, Spain, Portugal, and California.

PROPERTIES: Antiseptic, Antibacterial, Anti-inflammatory, Anti-spasmodic, Astringent, Carminative, Decongestant, Febrifuge, Hepatic, Hypotensive, Vermifuge and Vulnerary.

USES: Lemon is without doubt one of the most versatile of the oils and used in the right proportions has few contra-indications. Lemon essential oil neutralises typhus bacillus and staphylococcus in 5 minutes and diptheric bacillus in 20 minutes so it is a powerful bactericide. It is excellent for external wounds and infections and as a mouthwash for gum infections, gingivitis and mouth ulcers.

Lemon, along with a number of other widely used oils, is now being praised for its ability to combat food and environment-born pathogens. **See recipes.**

It helps with digestive problems, cleanses the blood and acts as a lymphatic decongestant so useful on cellulite, for obesity, high blood pressure, cholesterol, and arteriosclerosis.

It is worth noting that Lemon juice counteracts acidity in the body, citric acid neutralizes during digestion giving rise to carbonates and bicarbonates of potassium and calcium, which helps maintain alkalinity in the system.

Other uses include treatment for dandruff, PMT,

migraine, insect and snake bites.

Excellent for greasy skin problems.

Diabetes, cellulite and circulatory conditions like chilblains respond well to this oil.

Eases bronchial and sinus infections.

Use for sprains, muscular aches and pains and rheumatism.

TOP NOTE WHICH BLENDS WELL WITH: Geranium, Ylang Ylang, Lavender, Ginger, and Patchouli.

CAUTIONS: It does not keep well and careful storage is necessary. If it is not fresh it can irritate the skin. It should only be used in small proportions and is best mixed with another oil. It is phototoxic, so the skin should not be exposed to sunlight after use.

LEMONGRASS – CYMBOPOGON CITRATUS

Steam distilled from the fresh and partially dried grass, the oil in yellow/brown and has a strong lemon aroma. There are several varieties of lemongrass, but cymbopogon citratus is recommended for massage treatments. It is native to tropical Asia and is cultivated in India, Sri Lanka, Indonesia, Africa, Madagascar, the Seychelles, South and tropical North America.

PROPERTIES: Analgesic, Antidepressant, Anti-inflammatory, Antioxidant Antiseptic, Astringent, Bactericidal, Carminative, Deodorant, Febrifuge, Fungicidal, Galactagogic, Insecticide, Nervine, Sedative, and Tonic.

USES: As it acts as a sedative on the central nervous system it is useful for exhaustion and stress-related conditions. Can be used to relieve jet lag, clears headaches, and fatigue. It is calming too for the digestive system and particularly useful for gastro-enteritis and colitis

Used in traditional Indian medicine as a febrifuge. It can be used for infectious illness and fevers.

It is helpful for strengthening muscle tone, slack tissue, and poor circulation as it tones the muscles.

In very small proportions it is useful for congested and greasy skin conditions, acne, excessive perspiration and athletes foot.

Used extensively to flavour Eastern cooking. It is a mild

insect repellent.

TOP NOTE WHICH BLENDS WELL WITH:
Lavender, Basil, Rosemary, Jasmine, Palmarosa, Neroli and Ylang Ylang.

CAUTIONS: Use only in low dosage as it can be an irritant on sensitive skins. Do not use during pregnancy.

MANDARIN – CITRUS RETICULATA

Expressed from the peel of the fruit, it has a sweet, tangy aroma. It is golden yellow oil with blue/violet luminosity. Produced in South America mainly Brazil, China, Italy, California and the Mediterranean.

PROPERTIES: Antiseptic, Antifungal, Anti-spasmodic, Carminative, Chologogic, Cytophylactic, Digestive, Sedative, Tonic.

USES: A good tonic for the digestive system, it stimulates appetite and helps to regulate the metabolic processes. Aids in the secretion of bile as it has a stimulating effect on the liver.

It can be safely used on young children. It is useful for over-active or hyperactive youngsters or anyone who needs balancing and calming.

Nice for the elderly too as it has an uplifting quality and is therefore good for low spirits and convalescence.

Sedative to the nervous system and helps banish depression. Excellent for treating PMS particularly if mixed with Clary sage or Chamomile.

Mandarin is gentle oil and can be used safely during pregnancy; mixed with Lavender, Neroli or Chamomile in good base oil will prevent stretch marks.

TOP NOTE WHICH BLENDS WELL WITH:
Lavender, Chamomile, Black pepper, Petigrain, Rose and the Citrus oils.

CAUTION: May be phototoxic, so is best not used if going into strong sunlight. It is often adulterated and it deteriorates quickly

MARJORAM – ORIGANUM MAJORANA or MAJORANA HORTENSIS

Produced by steam distillation of the dried flowering herb, the oil is a pale yellow, mobile liquid, which darkens with age. It has a warm, woody aroma with a hint of camphor. There are several varieties of Marjoram and they are easily confused. Majorana is also known as knotted marjoram. Other varieties include O. onites (Pot marjoram), Thymus mastichino (Wild marjoram) and O. vulgare (Oregano), which is also a wild plant from which Oregano Essential oil is extracted. This will be studied separately as it has different properties.

PROPERTIES: Analgesic, Anaphrodisiac, Antiseptic, Antispasmodic, Antiviral, Bactericidal, Carminative, Cephalic, Cordial, Digestive, Diuretic, Emmenagogic, Expectorant, Hypotensive, Nervine, Sedative, Stomachic, Tonic, Vasodilator, Vulnerary.

USES: Well known as a culinary herb for flavouring, it has been used for centuries. It was constantly used for medicinal purposes in Ancient Greece and Southern Europe.

It is extremely helpful with chest infections, colds, asthma, sinusitis and earaches.

It is relaxing oil and mixed with Lavender or Sweet Orange will help insomnia.

For all stress related conditions, hypertension, heart conditions, headaches, migraine and nervous tension.

Used to help prevent bed-wetting and mixed with Mandarin and Lavender is excellent for hyperactivity in children.

It helps regulate the menstrual cycle and relieves painful periods. However it has the reputation for quelling sexual desire.

It is said to help regulate the thyroid.

It is good circulatory oil as it is warming, so therefore it will help with stiffness, rheumatism, arthritis, aches and pains, strains and bruising.

Mixed with Rosemary or Thyme it helps prevent falling hair and will keep the scalp healthy.

MIDDLE NOTE WHICH BLENDS WELL WITH: Lavender, Orange, Bergamot, Cedarwood, Rosemary, Cypress and Ylang Ylang.

CAUTIONS: It is best not to use this oil during the first 6 months of pregnancy mainly because of the variety of qualities available.

Over use could cause drowsiness.

MAY CHANG – LITSEA CUBEBA

Steam distilled from the fruits of a small tropical tree, the fruit is described as looking similar to peppers. It is chemically very like Lemongrass and Melissa and the therapeutic effects are similar to Lemongrass. It has a more truly lemon smell than either Melissa or Lemongrass but with a fruity tang. It belongs to the same family as the laurel, rosewood and cinnamon tree. Native to Asia especially China, it is cultivated in Taiwan and Japan.

PROPERTIES: Anti-depressant, Anti-inflammatory, Antiseptic, Astringent, Carminative, Cordial, Deodorant, Digestive, Galactagogic, Hypotensive, Insecticide, Stimulant, Stomachic, Tonic.

USES: Studies in China have confirmed May Chang's anti-arrhythmic properties. It is suggested that it may have a beneficial effect on coronary heart disease.

Also recognised for treating dysmenorrhoea, stomach cramps, lower back pain and headaches. It is an effective bronchodilator and can be used for problems of the respiratory system such as coughs, bronchitis and asthma.

As an anti-depressant, calming and balancing and it is most useful in treating cases of apathy, listlessness and indifference as it is a truly uplifting smell. Reduces anger.

Use it in skin care for its mild astringent properties, which can be helpful with acne and oily skin. May Chang oil

63

is also a very effective deodorant that helps to reduce excess perspiration, so added to a lotion it can be used to make an all-over body lotion. This oil may be mildly sensitising to a few individuals, but since it has a powerful aroma you only need tiny amounts, which reduces the likelihood of it being a problem for most people.

BLENDS WELL WITH: Almost all other oils.

CAUTIONS: Non-toxic and generally non-irritant.

OREGANO - OREGANUM VULGARE

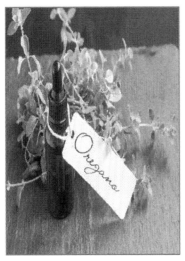

Used for over two thousand years, oregano essential oil is native to the Mediterranean region. It's amazing healing benefits were first discovered in Greece, where it was used as a topical anti-bacterial for the skin and for wounds. Growing wild in high altitude mountainous areas, it got its name, 'oregano,' or 'joy of the mountains.'

With over 40 different species available, it's important to note that the therapeutic benefits of oregano oil are only present in oil labelled as *Oreganum Vulgare.*

PROPERTIES: Anti-Allergenic, Antibacterial, Anti-Inflammatory, Antiviral, Analgesic, Antiseptic, Antifungal, Antihistamine, Antioxidant, Antidiabetic, Antiparasitical, Bechic, Decongestant, Digestive, Expectorant, Emmenagogic, Immuno-stimulant

USES: Research has shown that the carvacrol (phenol) in Oregano has promising potent healing properties and can fight several types of bacterial infections such as e.coli, candida albicans, salmonella, listeria, and staphylococcus aureus which is known to cause upper respiratory tract infections. Also useful for coughs, sinus blockage, asthma, croup, and bronchitis. Rubbed into the chest (suitably diluted) oregano oil breaks up mucus congestion.

Thymol, another phenol, has excellent antiseptic properties and is great for treating fungal infections, especially nail fungus and a contagious condition called tinea pedis, better known as Athlete's foot. It also helps protect against toxins and promotes healing.

Oregano essential oil is a must-have addition to your medicine cabinet. It is an excellent immunity booster. It also helps to aid digestion, fights candida, can alleviate severe allergy and menstrual symptoms,

Oregano is known as wild marjoram and is closely related to Marjoram (Oreganum marjorana). Because of the high content of carvacrol, Oregano oil has previously been scorned by Aromatherapists. But, in truth it offers a wide range of health benefits. It has demonstrated protective effects on the liver, antioxidant activity against bacteria and harmful organisms. In tiny dosages this oils has amazing health benefits.

Several research studies in The Global Health Centre in Texas have demonstrated the improving effect this oil has against breast, prostate, brain and lung cancer cells. Solution potency and application are major factors in all the research.

Other uses include treating menstrual cramps, rheumatoid arthritis, urinary tract disorders, headaches, and heart conditions. The oil of oregano is taken by mouth (tiny doses) for intestinal parasites, allergies, sinus pain, arthritis, cold and flu, earaches, and fatigue. Oregano oil does not kill off helpful probiotic bacteria the way that pharmaceutical antibiotics do.

It is applied to the skin for skin conditions including acne, athlete's foot, oily skin, dandruff, canker sores, warts, ringworm, rosacea, and psoriasis. Used for insect and spider bites, gum disease, toothaches, muscle pain, and varicose veins.

MIDDLE NOTE WHICH BLENDS WELL WITH: Lemon, May Chang, Lavender, Patchouli, Frankincense.

CAUTIONS: Do not apply so broken skin, sores or sensitive areas of the body. Could cause dermal irritation. Not to be used in Pregnancy at all.

PATCHOULI: POGOSTEMON CABLIN

Distilled from the leaves and shoots after they have been sun dried. The oil can vary from liquid and transparent to thick yellow/brown with a green tinge. It has an earthy, musty and pungent aroma. The oils are mainly produced in Sumatra, India, China, Japan, and the USA.

PROPERTIES: Antidepressant, Antiseptic, Antiviral, Anti-inflammatory, Aphrodisiac, Astringent, Diuretic, Cicatrisant, Nervine, Sedative, Tonic, Vulnerary.

USES: Patchouli has been used as a perfume for centuries. It is a natural fixative.

It is one of the oils that have a reputation as an Aphrodisiac perhaps because of its action on the Endocrine glands.

It is sedative in high doses and stimulating in small ones, so although it is a Base note it is perhaps better not used at night as the effect of stimulation or sedation, not only depends on the dose but also on the state of the individual.

It is recommended for many skin conditions such as herpes simplex, bedsores, impetigo, acne, burns, seborrhoea, eczema, and haemorrhoids. It is a skin rejuvenator, so is excellent for elderly skin.

It has an antidepressant effect and has been used in treatments of obesity, possibly because of reports (unsubstantiated) that it induces loss of appetite and because

68

it reduces water retention.

It has a balancing effect on the digestive system so can be used for both diarrhoea and constipation.

BLENDS WELL WITH: Bergamot, Oregano, Clove, Lavender, Rose, Clary Sage, Cedarwood, Black Pepper and Lemongrass.

CAUTIONS:
This oil is often adulterated so get to know it well.

PEPPERMINT - MENTHA PIPERITA

Steam distilled from the flowering herb, with a highly penetrating odour. Produced mainly in France, Bulgaria, Russia, USA, Italy, Hungary, Morocco, China, and the UK. There are a number of mint species. Mentha Spicata is the only one recommended for home use.

PROPERTIES: Anaesthetic, Analgesic, Antigalactigogic, Anti-inflammatory, Antiseptic, Antispasmodic, Astringent, Antiviral, Carminative, Cephalic, Chologogic, Cordial, Decongestant, Digestive, Emmenagogic, Expectorant, Febrifuge, Hepatic, Nervine, Stimulant, Stomachic, Sudorific, Vasoconstrictor, Vermifuge.

USES: Peppermint is one of the most versatile essential oils. There are few issues that it can't help. Possibly the most fascinating aspect of peppermint is that recent research suggests that it is literally antibiotic resistant. According to an article published in the journal *Phytomedicine* in 2013, 'Reduced usage of antibiotics could be employed as a treatment strategy to decrease the adverse effects and possibly to reverse the beta-lactam antibiotic resistance, due to the powerful effects of peppermint oil.'

Antibiotic-resistant bacteria have been a major cause of concern for many who are simply ruining their health by taking too many of these dangerous drugs.

Excellent oil for mental fatigue, anger, hysteria and

nervous tension.

Peppermint is useful for relaxing the stomach so can be used for acute problems of diarrhoea and constipation, nausea, flatulence, gallstones and food poisoning. Its cooling and pain relieving actions make it useful for migraine headaches, toothache, aching limbs, joints and neuralgia. It is useful in fever cases and as a decongestant for colds and flu, sinus or mucus problems. Used for asthma because it is antispasmodic, but not inhaled directly. Also for acne, dermatitis, ringworm, and scabies used in small proportion it will help the irritation and infection.

Lovely for aching feet.

MIDDLE NOTE WHICH BLENDS WELL: Lavender, Marjoram, Ylang Ylang, Oregano, Patchouli and Orange

CAUTIONS: Dosage should always be small as it can cause skin sensitivity. Use in infusers and apply locally. Best avoided by nursing mothers since it could discourage the flow of milk.

ROSEMARY - ROSEMARINUS OFFICINALIS

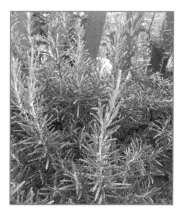 Distilled from the flowering tops, stems, and leaves of the plant. The oil is colourless to pale yellow/green. It should smell like camphor with a hint of incense and honey. The best oils come from North Africa, mainly Tunisia, but other good oils are produced in Mediterranean countries and Yugoslavia.

PROPERTIES: Analgesic, Antidepressant, Antiseptic, Antispasmodic, Astringent, Carminative, Cephalic, Chologogic, Cicatrisant, Decongestant, Diuretic, Emmenogogue, Hepatic, Hypertensive, Nervine, Stimulant, Stomachic, Sudorific, Tonic, and Vulnerary.

USES: In Ancient Greece Rosemary was a symbol of love and death. It has been used for centuries in hair and beauty products. It has a tonic effect on dark hair and it helps it to retain its colour. It even has a history of stimulating hair growth.

Rosemary is useful for treating fatigue and headaches as it has the ability to enliven the brain cells. It helps relieve colds, and flu and over tired muscles.

One amazing healing effect of Rosemary that many people are unaware of is its ability to normalize blood

72

pressure. In one of the few human studies evaluating this phenomenon, researchers from the Universidad Complutense de Madrid took 32 hypotensive patients and measured how their dangerously low blood pressure fared under Rosemary essential oil treatments for 72 weeks with astounding results. In addition to observing that Rosemary could raise blood pressure to normal limits in a vast majority of the volunteers, it was discovered that overall mental and physical quality of life was drastically improved, which highlights the far-reaching healing effects that this ancient oil has on health and wellness.

Used for centuries to improve everything from memory and brain function to relieving the common aches and pains of arthritis, joint pains and strains. Rosemary is also excellent for digestive problems and is particularly good for constipation, as it seems to stimulate peristalsis.

Helps relieve congestion generally in the body so helps with cellulite, fluid retention, and obesity.

MIDDLE NOTE WHICH BLENDS WELL WITH: Lavender, Patchouli, Neroli, Mandarin, Black pepper, Cinnamon.

CAUTIONS: There are many different varieties of Rosemary oil and it best to stick to the officinalis as the borneol, cineole and verbone are a different chemical make-up. Because Rosemary is highly stimulating it may not be suitable for people with high blood pressure and should be avoided by epileptics. It is best avoided during pregnancy.

TEA TREE - MELALEUCA ALTERNIFOLIA

Distilled from the leaves of the tree, the oil is a very pale yellow green. It has a spicy, antiseptic aroma. It is only grown in New South Wales, Australia.

PROPERTIES: Antifungal, Antibacterial, Anti-inflammatory, Antiseptic, Antiviral, Cicatrisant, Cytophylactic, Decongestant, and Vulnerary.

USES: Because this oil is 11-12 times more antiseptic than carbolic acid or phenol it is effective against a range of bacterial, viral and fungal conditions. It is used widely in disinfectant, toothpaste, and gargles. It has the added advantage of being both hypoallergenic and non-toxic.

It is useful in treating colds and flu and alleviates sore throats, tonsillitis, and gum disease. It eases bronchitis and congestion.

It calms diarrhoea and relieves gastro-enteritis. It is useful in treating candida albicans. and invaluable for treating complaints of the genito-urinary system such as thrush, trichomonal, cystitis and vaginitis. Is effective for skin problems, particularly boils, acne, infected wounds and burns or fungal problems (including athletes foot and jock itch).
It is also an extremely effective insect repellent

Although Tea Tree is relatively new oil in terms of Aromatherapy the natives of Australia have used it for centuries. This oil has been extensively researched and

74

documented. In 1980 it was subjected to stringent testing and it was found that a solution 4 parts Essential oil to 1000 parts water, used against virulent organisms such as staphylococus aureas and candida albicans showed that after testing on the 7th, 21st and 35th days there was no growth detected in the organism. This suggests that when the body is threatened, Tea Tree has the ability to support the Immune response.

TOP TO MIDDLE NOTE WHICH BLENDS WELL WITH: Other Melaleucas, Geranium, Lavender, Ylang Ylang, Cinnamon, Marjoram, Orange, Bergamot, Eucalyptus. Does not blend well with the spice oils.

CAUTIONS: Slight possibility of irritation on sensitive skin or prolonged use.

THYME – THYMUS VULGARIS

There are hundreds of varieties of Thyme but vulgaris is known as common or garden thyme and grows everywhere in Europe, Asia and North Africa. Although it has a harsh smell mixed with oils such as Lavender, Geranium, Ylang Ylang or Mandarin it achieves a sweetness.

PROPERTIES: Antirheumatic, Antiseptic, Antispasmodic, Astringent, Aphrodisiac, Bechic, Cardiac, Carminative, Cicatrisant, Diuretic, Emmenagogic, Expectorant, Hypertensive, Insecticide, Nervine, Rubifacient, Stimulant, Tonic, Vermifuge.

USES: Traditionally used for protection against disease and infection. It is highly antiseptic. Thyme has been used in many ways over the centuries particularly for the nervous system, for depression and to re-establish strength during convalescence. Hippocrates wrote about thyme in over 400 of his medical recipes. It was used as a 'strewing herb' and was included in posies carried by judges, doctors and kings to protect them in public places.

It is an aid to protect the nerves and activate brain cells, helping memory and concentration, depression, low spirits, exhaustion and trauma.

The respiratory system responds well and it can be used effectively with whooping cough and fever.

For pain relief, mix with the other anti inflammatory

and analgesic oils.

It is immune supporting and it activates the white blood cells so strengthening the body's resistance to invading organisms.

BLENDS WELL WITH: Bergamot, Juniper, Mandarin, Rosemary and the flower oils.

CAUTIONS: Because there are so many chemotypes it is difficult to know what constituents are in your oil. Buy the best you can afford and use sparingly. It is invaluable oil and has had so many traditional uses that are not to be ignored. It can cause dermal irritation and should not be used on mucus membrane.

TURMERIC – CURCUMA LONGA

Derived from the plant's tuberous rhizomes or underground roots. Turmeric has a lengthy history as a medicine, spice and colouring agent, and is an extremely impressive natural health agent — one that has some of the most promising anticancer effects around. It also contains vitamins, phenols and other alkaloids.

Turmeric has a long history of medicinal use in South Asia. Topically speaking, turmeric essential oil is traditionally used as an antiseptic and in natural skin care to discourage acne and facial hair in women.

PROPERTIES: Anti-allergic, Antibacterial, Antibiotic, Anticonvulsant, Anti-inflammatory, Antimicrobial, Antifungal, Antioxidant, Anti-parasitic, Antiviral, Relaxant, Energising, Vermifuge.

USES: Turmeric health benefits are truly amazing, ranging from working as a potential cancer-fighting food to an essential oil for depression. This oil is considered a strong relaxant and balancer. Studies have shown that curcumin in turmeric successfully reduces the overall symptoms of depression and also works as an anti-anxiety agent when taken over a period of eight weeks.

According to Ayurvedic medicine, it will support the imbalance of Kapha body type.

The essential oil of turmeric is reported to help fight

against leukaemia, breast and colon cancer.

Turmeric oil has been shown to stimulate regeneration of cells in the brain, making it effective at improving neurologic diseases like Parkinson's, Alzheimer's, spinal cord injury and stroke.

Turmeric is well known in the holistic health world for its ability to improve liver health. The liver can greatly benefit from turmeric essential oil's protective and anti-inflammatory abilities. Using the oil topically helps reduce pain, soothe joint and muscle aches and reduce inflammation and stiffness related to rheumatoid arthritis and osteoarthritis.

Turmeric essential oil is more often used topically but can also be used internally if you're using very high-quality oil and use small dosages (1 drop of essential oil).

BASE NOTE WHICH BLENDS WELL WITH: Ginger, Cinnamon, Grapefruit, Ylang Ylang and Lavender.

CAUTION: As with all essential oils, turmeric essential oil should not be used undiluted. Don't take turmeric oil internally unless you're working with a qualified and expert practitioner. Do not use if you're pregnant, nursing, taking medication or being treated for any health condition. Turmeric essential oil is very potent, and a little goes a long way.

One negative turmeric side effect is its ability to stain clothes and skin, whether you use the spice or the oil. Turmeric essential oil is yellow just like the spice and can easily and permanently dyes your clothing. It can also temporarily leave your skin looking yellow. It might take a few washings, but the colour will leave your skin. Wiping the stained area with coconut oil or lemon juice can help remove any skin staining more quickly.

Turmeric essential oil, like many other essential oils, also can make your skin more sensitive to UV light so use caution.

YLANG YLANG – CANANGA ODORATA

Steam distilled from the flowers (the name means flower of flowers in Malay) the oil is colourless to pale yellow. This essential oil is collected at various stages and graded accordingly. Each successive collection of oil produces differing grades and containing a wide array of chemical constituents.

It is sold in various grades: Extra, 1, 2, 3, Complete.

Extra Grade: Regarded by many as containing the finest notes from the distillation process, the first collection after an hour or two of steam distillation. Contains roughly 30 different chemical constituents, it is usually the most expensive.

Grade I – III: As the steam distillation process continues, essential oil collections are taken every few hours, which make up less potent and less expensive. Oils in descending order: Grade I, then II and finally III.

Complete: Represents the whole distillate encompassing all the collections from the entire distillation process. This synergy oil offers maximum fragrance potency. It has a heavy sweet aroma.

PROPERTIES: Antiseptic, Antidepressant, Antidiabetic, Anti-inflammatory, Aphrodisiac, Carminative, Insecticidal, Hypotensive, and Sedative.

USES: This oil is best known for its ability to reduce heart rate (tachycardia) and rapid breathing (hyperpnoea). It is excellent to use in cases of shock, anger, fear, overwork and frustration (including sexual) or anxiety and it helps reduce high blood pressure.

Its qualities are well known in helping with sexual problems such as impotence and frigidity. Traditionally used to enhance sexual function, inhaling Ylang Ylang oil is actually only proven to reduce the anxiety related to sex. This is not to say that our ancestors were misled in using it for sexual enhancement, but just that there is little modern research to substantiate it.

Either way, using Ylang Ylang oil can help enhance your sexual experience, so I give it thumbs up!

It is oil that is widely used in the perfume and cosmetic industry and is known to be a scalp tonic. In the Victorian age, the oil was used in a popular hair treatment, Macassar oil, due to its stimulating effect on the scalp, encouraging hair growth.

Mixed with coconut oil it was used by the natives of the Philippine islands to protect their hair and their skin when they swam. They called it borri-borri and also used it to avoid the bites of snakes and insects.

In addition to the sedative properties mentioned above via inhalation, studies also suggest that topical application is exceptionally calming as well. The results of one 2006 study discovered that simply massaging a 20% solution of Ylang Ylang oil in sweet almond oil over the abdomen for 5 minutes, then wrapped with plastic film to prevent evaporation resulted in a significant decrease of blood pressure and a lowering of skin temperature, which is an indication of muscle relaxation and, therefore, a decrease in sympathetic nervous system functioning.

Ylang Ylang has had many uses in traditional medicine ranging from a skin tonic, to helping to relieve insect bite irritation, to treating more serious health concerns like malaria, asthma, gout, and digestive issues.

BASE NOTE WHICH BLENDS WELL WITH: Lemon, May Chang and Bergamot, Lemongrass, Lemon, Eucalyptus, Lavender and Bergamot. Most help reduce the slightly sweet sickly aroma that can sometimes induce nausea and headaches.

CAUTIONS: In excess can cause headaches and nausea. Should not be used on inflamed skin conditions.

IN THE KITCHEN

Harmful cleaning chemicals are effective and fast but highly toxic to everything, whereas using essential oils for cleaning will not be fast but they will disinfect and deodorise just as efficiently and smell natural and real.

GENERAL CLEANING.

Many essential oils have anti-fungal properties so are useful for areas where food is stored. The anti-bacterial properties of oils like **Lavender, Lemon, Ravensara, Peppermint, Tea Tree and Lemongrass** make them ideal for cleaning areas like worktops, waste bins and pet beds.

Being natural chemicals they will not contaminate the waterways into which so much of our daily waste is routinely deposited. The tiny quantities required means they are safe and also make them highly economical.

There is a great deal of research being done into the value of these lovely products and we know that good quality oils, used properly, can make sure that your home is germ and bacteria free, fragrant and clean.

A few ideas:

Fridge cleaning, Worktops, Floors: 1 drop of **Lavender, Lemongrass, Tea tree, Oregano, Lemon or Geranium** and 1 drop of **Grapefruit** in 1 pint of water.

Waste bins: Add 2 drops of **Tea Tree, Lavender, Lemon,**

Cedarwood or Lemongrass to a damp cloth.

Pet Care: Clean plastic and wicker baskets with a damp cloth onto which you have added 2 drops of **Lemon, Lavender, Cedarwood or Tea Tree**. When washing your pets bedding add 4 drops of oil to the final rinse cycle. For keeping pets clean and free from tics and fleas, sprinkle a few drops of **Juniper, Cedarwood, Oregano, Lavender,** or **Tea Tree** on their bedding or use 4-5 drops in their bath water. Mixed with water or alcohol the oils can be rubbed into or brushed through your pet's coat.

Airing cupboard: Fold a tissue or a cotton wool pad and add 4 drops of **Cedarwood, Lavender, Geranium, Sandalwood, Patchouli** or **Ylang Ylang**. Base notes obviously last the longest. This can be placed between towels, sheets and duvet covers.
Make a blend you really like and use in all your drawers and cupboards. Incidentally most of these oils are moths and insect repellents too.

Fresh Air Spray: A great idea is to make your own spritzer spray. To 100 mls of water add 10 drops of witch hazel, 10 drops of grain alcohol and 6-10 drops of essential oils of your choice. Put into a pump action spray bottle and you have a chemical free way of making your home smell fragrant as well as keeping it germ free.
Shake well before use.

Smelly footwear: Put 2-3 drops of **Lemongrass, May Chang, Oregano** or **Lavender** onto an unused dry teabag and leave in the offending footwear.

ADD FLAVOUR TO EVERYDAY RECIPES: All the citrus oil and floral oils are great in puddings, marzipan, sweet breads, mousse, crêpes, custards, ice cream, fruit pies, icing and cakes. Try 1 drop of **Cinnamon, Clove, Orange, Lemon, Rose, Peppermint** or **Ginger.**

In one pint of carrot soup: add 3 drops of **Mandarin** to a teaspoon olive oil and stir into soup a minute before serving. Others that can be included in vegetable and meat dishes are **Rosemary, Thyme, Turmeric, Oregano, Orange, Ginger, Lemon, Basil, and Coriander.** One drop of essential oil equates to one teaspoon of herbs so use carefully.

ESSENTIAL OILS FOR CHILDREN

Most oils can be used safely and happily on children of all ages. But, it is dosage that is important. Always use half the recommended doses as for adults but it is best to use a sliding scale according to age and growth. From babyhood to adolescence, children respond really well to aromatherapy, partly because they have no preformed expectations and because young bodies have excellent powers of recuperation and healing.

You do not need to be a trained masseuse to rub away your child's pain or discomfort. It is something that comes quite naturally: to sooth by physical touch or stroking. This sort of body contact can be exceptionally bonding for parent and child. Gentle massage with good base oil and the safe essential oils is extremely beneficial and soothing for parent and child alike.

Regular use of essential oils in the home is a very effective form of preventative medicine. Using a diffuser or simple application is best but in their bath or a few drops on their pillow can work wonders.

Local application is recommended in the case of pain or over activity. For example, when your child wakes up scared after a nightmare, apply **Cedarwood** or **Lavender** oil in a few drops of **Almond** oil to the bottom of his/her feet to help promote a peaceful settled feeling.

The citrus oils **Orange, Grapefruit. Lemon** and **Mandarin** are all excellent for children. **Lavender, Rose.**

Roman Chamomile, Eucalyptus Radiata, Geranium, Tea Tree and **Peppermint** are all oils that can be used safely.

Read carefully the way oils are described and you will quickly be able to decide which are best.

Below is a list of single oils to try in specific situations and the right proportions.
Asthma: **Frankincense.** Bed-wetting: **Marjoram.** Constipation: **Rosemary.** Cradle cap: **Geranium.** Cuts, grazes and bruises: **Tea Tree.** Diarrhoea: **Ginger.** Eczema: **Chamomile.** Fretfulness: **Lavender.** Sniffles and colds: **Eucalyptus Radiata.**

ADHD (Attention Deficit Hyperactivity Disorder).

At times, most children have trouble paying attention, listening, or sitting still. But those with ADHD have trouble with these things almost all the time.

ADHD is a medical condition that affects self-control and focus. It can also make them more fidgety than others of their age so the calming oils can be used in a diffuser to help concentration and attention. Massage is also recommended but because it is difficult to contain a child with this syndrome, short treatments are best.

All of the relaxing oils are useful. Try **Vetivert** and **Mandarin** in a diffuser and **Lavender** and **Marjoram** in a bath or massage.

Disabilty

All children are different and those with disabilities each have their own specific needs. Many respond extremely well to massage and sensory stimulus and particularly to essential oils. Use exactly as you would for anyone else, being careful of dosage and choice of oils. All of the citrus oils are particularly helpful as well as the oils for specific problems like relaxation, mobility and pain. Choose with care. Decide whether relaxing or stimulating oils are needed and if it is not possible to massage the torso give a foot, head or hand massage. Gentle repetitive movements are the best and most therapeutic.

Never attempt to treat serious illness. Consult your GP if your child is running an extremely high temperature, is badly hurt or has convulsions.

RECIPES

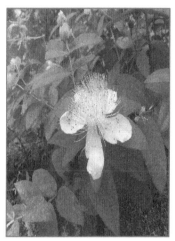

The following are a few example recipes that show just how versatile the oils really are. The mixes of essential oils are generally a Top, Middle and Base note, which give a balanced treatment. The Carrier oils are the oily base oils into which we mix the essential oils. Because they are a compound of glycerol and fatty acids they are integrated and absorb the essential oil molecules. They should be carefully chosen as many have therapeutic properties themselves. They act as balancing and stabilising agents. Cold pressed is best, and they should have little or no smell. Grapeseed, Coconut, Almond, Sunflower, Jojoba and Hypericum are all good examples.

ALLERGIES: Oils that are anti-allergenic, anti-inflammatory help reduce the way the body reacts to allergens such as pollen, mould and other airborne irritants that can cause inflammation in the airways. **Lavender, Lemon, Chamomile, Peppermint, Turmeric** and **Oregano** can be used in a diffuser or as a mix, in a bath, for inhalation or for a massage.

Therapeutic-grade oregano oil contains carvacrol, which has anti-inflammatory properties, and rosmarinic acid, a natural constituent that can help reduce swelling and is effective in treating allergic reactions. Both of these active components found in oregano essential oil can help relieve allergy symptoms like sneezing, congestion, and itching. Chamomile is anti-inflammatory and calming. Peppermint is antispasmodic and carminative in tiny amounts. Lavender is a balancing oil and Lemon is decongestant.

ANXIETY: Any of the **Citrus oils, Clary Sage, Bergamot, Lavender, Chamomile, Rose, Ylang Ylang, Neroli** and **Frankincense,** suitably diluted can be used as local application, massaged into the chest and lower spine daily. For a full body massage try 2 drops **Mandarin**, 2 drops of **Chamomile** and 2 drops of **Ylang Ylang** in 12 to14 mls of base oil. Use daily in a diffuser.
Other considerations: Learn some deep breathing and relaxation exercises. Self care.

ARTHRITIS: In most cases of arthritis the body is not eliminating uric acid and waste products efficiently. Stress, poor diet and environmental pollution all cause toxic waste in the body. There are many different symptoms and varieties of arthritis. Some are caused by infection. It is often the joints used most heavily, either in sport, physical occupation, incorrect posture or dealing with being overweight that are affected. Inflammation occurs, circulation becomes impaired. Distortion of the joint causes stiffness and pain.

All of the anti-inflammatory oils will help. They include **Oregano, Jasmin, Eucalyptus Radiata, Lavender, Lemon,**

May Chang, Patchouli, Pine, Thyme, Ginger, Tea Tree, Marjoram, Chamomile, Peppermint, Rosemary, Turmeric and **Ylang Ylang.**

There are so many combinations here.

Try **I drop Oregano, 2 drops Ginger** and **2 drops of Marjoram** with 5 mls of lotion, almond oil or cream to massage into affected areas.

Alternatively, 1 drop **Peppermint**, 1 drop **Turmeric,** 2 drops **Chamomile** and 2 drops **Rosemary** in base oil for a full body massage.

Combine 3 drops **Lavender,** 3 drops **Tea Tree** and 3 drops of **Marjoram** into a teaspoon of oil or milk and add to a warm bath. Add Epsom salts for extra detoxification.

Other considerations: Diet, Exercise, Warmth. Nutrition should include lots of vegetables, a reduction of dairy products, red meat, smoked and refined products and acid producing foods.

ASTHMA: Although steam inhalation it is not recommended for asthmatics, direct inhalation at the time of crisis can be beneficial. The Antispasmodic oils **Hyssop, Eucalyptus. Rosemary, Oregano, Basil, Marjoram, Frankincense, Ravensara, Clary Sage,** and **Cedarwood** are best.

Other considerations: Stress, chemicals, environment. Diet: reduce dairy products, processed foods, colas, sugar, and caffeine.

ATHLETES FOOT: Soak the affected foot for 15-20 minutes in a solution of warm water with 4 drops of any of the antifungal oils, **Oregano, Tea Tree, Bergamot,**

Eucalyptus, Geranium, Thyme, Lavender. Do this twice a day for best results. You can also add ½ a cup of Epsom salts as this will help to relax your muscles.

Athlete's foot is commonly spread in changing rooms, gyms, swimming pools and areas where people with infected feet walk around barefoot. As a precaution, rub your feet with a few drops of oregano oil combined with carrier oil such as almond or calendula prior to visiting these places, or keep a few small cotton balls soaked in the same blend in your shoes to prevent an infection.

BLOOD PRESSURE:
High: **Ylang Ylang, Lavender, Clary Sage, May Chang, Marjoram** and **Juniper.**
Low: **Rosemary, Lavender, Thyme Neroli.**

BRONCHITIS: There are many oils that help but the following combination can be rubbed in the chest and back several times daily to relieve the symptoms.

2 drops **Eucalyptus Globulus,** 2 drops **Marjoram**, 2 drops **Ginger**, 1 drop **Clove** and 1 drop **Oregano** mixed into 15 mls plain body lotion or Almond base oil.

Use a diffuser with a similar combination of essential oils.

CANDIDA: Take sublingually. For internal yeast infections, add 2-3 drops of **Oregano or Tea Tree or Myrrh** oil to an edible carrier oil such as olive or coconut oil and take it sublingually (under your tongue). Swish the blend under the tongue for a minute or so giving it time to absorb into your blood, and then spit it out into a tissue. Repeat 2-3 times a day.

Other considerations: Eliminate sugar from the diet and take probiotics.

CELLULITE: Use in a massage and in the bath. Combine **Grapefruit, Juniper Berry, and Patchouli.**

Other considerations: Massage, Diet, Water, Skin Brushing.

CIRCULATION: Geranium, Nutmeg, Ginger, Black Pepper, Grapefruit, Clove and **Fennel** are good for circulatory problems, chilblains, Reynard's Disease and leg cramps. Massage will be the best treatment as it is a passive way of exercising and it improves the blood flow around the body.

COLD SORES: Bergamot, Tea Tree, Lemon Grass, Oregano, Geranium, and **Patchouli.** Put a single drop of any of these oils onto a cotton bud and dab onto sore twice a day.

Other considerations: General immune health.

COLDS & FLU: If you feel the symptoms of flu coming on and want a natural go-to remedy to stave off falling sick, there are several essential oils that can help.

In your bath: 10 or 12 drops of **Ravensara, Eucalyptus,** and **Tea Tree** added to a full bath of water. It is a good idea to mix oils with a little carrier oil or milk so that they will distribute into the bath water.

Steam inhalation: Add a few drops of **Oregano, Eucalyptus,**
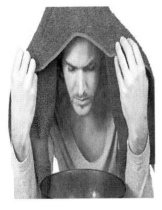
Marjoram or **Tea Tree** oil to a bowl of boiling water, place a towel over your head and breathe in the powerful vapours for 5-10 minutes. The moist steam helps to loosen and drain mucus in the nasal passages and the antibacterial properties of the oil help to fight infections and relieve cold symptoms.

Add several drops of **Oregano, Eucalyptus, Lavender,** and **Peppermint** into your diffuser and breathe in the medicinal vapours.

Inhale directly: A deep sniff of **Rosemary, Oregano, Lemon, Eucalyptus** oil directly from the bottle is a great pick-me-up and can help open up the airways.

Sore throat: Add 1 drop of **Tea Tree or Oregano oil** to a small glass of warm water and gargle with the blend. Swish around really well as oil and water do not thoroughly combine. The antibacterial properties of the oil will help to ward off bacteria and the anti-inflammatory properties will help to soothe an aching throat.

Take sublingually: Add 2 drops of **Oregano, Lemon** or **Tea Tree oil** to a tablespoon of edible carrier oil such as olive or coconut oil and take it sublingually (under your tongue). Swish around for a minute, and then spit it out into a tissue. Do not spit into sink as the coconut oil will harden and clog your pipes. Repeat twice daily.

CONSTIPATION: Any of the **Citrus** oils and most of the **Spice** oils, **Peppermint, Black Pepper, Patchouli, Hyssop, Fennel, Mandarin, Marjoram, Ginger, Juniper Berry** and **Chamomile** all help.

Mix 3 drops **Mandarin**, 2 drops **Black Pepper** and 2 drops **Ginger** or 2 drops **Rosemary**, 2 drops **Caraway** and 3 drops **Patchouli** (7 drops to the 10mls of base oil) with 10 mls base oils or cream and massage into abdomen twice a day. *Other considerations:* Exercise. Diet, such as fibre intake, fruit and vegetables. Drink plenty of water. Habit (Try to take time to sit and eliminate at the same time every day)

CRAMP: **Basil, Lavender, Marjoram, Rosemary, Peppermint, Ginger, and Geranium.** Dilute 2 or 3 drops with 3mls of base oil or cream and massage affected areas. *Other considerations:* Exercise, relaxation, mineral deficiency.

CYSTITIS: Mix 10 drops of any of the following or a combination making up 10 drops in 12 mls of base oils and rub into pelvic area 3 or 4 times daily. **Clary Sage, Mandarin, Chamomile, Geranium, Lavender, Peppermint, Rosemary, Fennel, Neroli, Rose.** *Other considerations:* Drink lots of water. No caffeine, fizzy drinks, alcohol and fruit juices except Cranberry juice. Eat bananas, blueberries and melon. Refrain from sex.

DANDRUFF: Add 10 drops **Rosemary (Brunettes)**, **Cedarwood, Oregano, Marjoram, Ylang Ylang, Thyme, Lavender or Lemon (Blondes)** into your final rinse.

DEPRESSION: **May Chang, Geranium, Neroli, Frankincense, Lavender, Orange, Grapefruit, Chamomile, Marjoram, Ylang Ylang.** Use singly or in combination for massage or a diffuser.

Other considerations: Lifestyle, diet, exercise / relaxation, vitamin supplements.

DIABETES: Diabetes mellitus is a disease that prevents your body from properly using the energy from the food you eat. When sugar leaves the bloodstream and enters the cells, the blood sugar level is lowered. Without insulin, or the 'key,' sugar cannot get into the body's cells for use as energy. Too much sugar in the blood is called 'hyperglycaemia' (high blood sugar) or diabetes. In the bath or in a massage essential oils can help you control your blood sugar. Oils for use with diabetics include: **Cinnamon, Geranium, Clary Sage, Eucalyptus, Juniper, Ginger, Lemon Ylang Ylang** and **Vetivert.**

Other considerations: Diet (eat porridge for breakfast as it helps slow absorption of sugars. Sprinkle with Cinnamon.) Improve your intake of foods containing Zinc, Potassium and Chromium.

EAR ACHE & INFECTION: Add 2-3 drops of **Oregano, Tea Tree, Chamomile, Lavender or Basil** oil with 2-3 drops of a carrier oil such as **Jojoba** or **Coconut oil** and massage it around the outside of the ear. Be careful not to get it inside the ear canal. The oil will permeate the skin and absorb into the tissues and help alleviate pain and throbbing in the ear.

Alternatively crush a clove of garlic and soak in warm olive oil for about 15 minutes. Strain and put a few drops in affected ear.

ENDOMETRIOSIS: A condition where the tissue that lines the womb (endometrium) is found outside the womb, such as in the ovaries and fallopian tubes. There are treatments that can help but it can be a painful long-term problem. Endometriosis mainly affects girls and women of childbearing age. To help relieve the pain try any combination of 10 drops of essential oils to 12 mls carrier oil or lotion applied twice a day to whole stomach area. **Clary Sage, May Chang, Cypress, Geranium, Lavender** and **Fennel.**

EYE INFECTION: Diluted in 10 mls **Almond** or **Grapeseed** 2 drops **Clary Sage,** and 2 drops **Chamomile German.** Use eyebath and swill around eyes. Wait until eyes are clear before moving.

FATIGUE: Use in a burner of diffuser or direct inhalation from the bottle. **Basil, Bergamot, Lemongrass, May Chang, Black Pepper, Rosemary, Peppermint, Eucalyptus, Clove, Orange, Lemon, Neroli, Lavender, Geranium, Roman Chamomile.**

FIBROMYALGIA: A chronic condition that characteristically causes pain all over the body, including muscle and joint pain, profound fatigue, disturbed sleep and a myriad of other symptoms. Any of the analgesic oils help and each person finds a different combination.

Try the following recipe: 10mls **Coconut oil** and 15 mls of **Shea Butter.** Fully melt the coconut oil and Shea butter in a non-stick pan over low heat. Allow to cool for a few minutes. Add 5 drops of **Ginger,** 5 drops **Vetivert** and 10 drops of **Lemongrass** and whisk. Pour the oil into an amber glass jar, using a stainless steel funnel to prevent spillage. Use locally or for massage twice daily.

GUMS AND BAD BREATH: 1 drop **Tea Tree** on your toothpaste when brushing. Also effective **Frankincense, Myrrh, Clove** and **Ginger.** A really good **mouthwash** can be made with 250mls cheap brandy or vodka to which you add 30 drops **Thyme**, 30 drops **Peppermint**, 10 drops **Oregano**, 10 drop **Fennel.** Shake well before adding 2 or 3 teaspoons of the mix to a half a cup of water.

GOUT: All the anti-inflammatory and analgesic oils including **Frankincense, Rosemary, Basil, Thyme, Geranium, Ginger**, and **Chamomile.** Massage into affected areas, 2 drops of 3 of the above essential oils (6 drops) into half teaspoon of olive oil.

Other considerations: Reduce alcohol and meat laden foods. Eat cherries! High in Vitamin C and fibre they reduce uric acid in the body. So does other fruit but cherries are purported to increase the production of anthocyanin in the bloodstream, which does help gout. Well worth a try!

HAEMORROIDS: Bathe sore areas with the following blend: Mix **2 drops Patchouli, 10 drop Myrrh, 5 drops Cypress.** Put only 4 drops of this blend in 5mls of cream or oil apply to anal area with a piece of cotton wool 3-4 times a day.

HAIR TONIC: Mix 10 drops of **Juniper** or **Thyme** with 8 drops **Rosemary** or **Lavender** and 7 Drops **Cedarwood** into 50 mls **Olive oil**. Massage into head and hair, wrap in a towel and leave for at least two hours. Add mild shampoo and wash as normal.

HANGOVER: **Grapefruit, May Chang, Rosemary.** Add a few drops to a bath or 2 drops of each in a diffuser.
Other considerations – Dependency, relaxation, stress.

HAY FEVER: The oils that have the strongest effect on hay fever include: **Ravensara – Hyssop – Eucalyptus radiata – Rosemary – Clary Sage – Cedarwood – Thyme – Frankincense.** Use in a diffuser in the house or make a mix to sniff.

In the winter months and during high pollen counts, take a spoonful of locally produced honey. It is said to help desensitise you to pollen although there is little evidence to support this. It's worth a try!

HEADACHE & MIGRAINE: **Lemon, Rosemary, Peppermint** in a diffuser or a small amount diluted and rubbed into temples sometimes helps.

Other considerations – Spine, exercise, digestion, diet, fresh air, stress.

HERPES: Mix 3-4 drops of **Oregano** essential oil with 1 tablespoon of a carrier such as **Coconut oil**, a natural anti-viral. Apply the blend onto the spine as the herpes virus lays dormant in the spinal column and usually infects the cerebrospinal fluid. This is the case with other viruses as well, so essentially doing this daily can help protect you from other viral attacks.

IBS: **Oregano, Rosemary Ginger. Lavender. Orange, Peppermint, Chamomile German** and **Marjoram** are all helpful. Take any three and add 3 drops of each to 10 mls of oil, cream or lotion and apply to abdomen 3 or 4 times a day.

IMMUNITY BOOSTING: Mix 3 drops of each **Cinnamon, Clove, Eucalyptus, Orange, Lemon and Rosemary** = 18 drops, with 40 mls Coconut oil or 40 mls cream base. Mix well. Rub unto lower spine and throat morning and evening.

Other Immune boosting oils are as follows: **Bergamot, Cedarwood, Cypress, Roman Chamomile, Frankincense, Geranium, Ginger, Lemongrass, Ravensara, Manuka, Neroli, Thyme** and **Tea Tree.**

All oils that are antioxidant (because that indicates a healing effect) are helpful to the immune system and act as a preventative medicine against infections and degenerative illnesses. Antioxidants act as scavengers, searching for free radicals to stop and prevent inflammation and damage. Use 10 drops of your favourite mix in a bath

INSOMNIA: Clary Sage, Lavender (angustifolia only), Rose, Vetivert, and Roman Chamomile. Use in a diffuser.
Other considerations: Stress, stimulants, diet, exercise, fresh air, relaxation.

LIP CARE: For sore lips or just general protection in harsh weather. Mix 1 teaspoon of beeswax with one teaspoon of honey. Add one teaspoons of almond oil and melt together. Whip and when cool add the contents of one capsule of Vit E and add 5 drops of any of the following: **Geranium, Rose, Lavender, Chamomile or Lemon.**

For **Cold Sores** add 4 drops of **Peppermint**, 4 drops of **Tea Tree** and 4 drops of **Bergamot** and apply at least 3 times a day.

MASTITIS: **Frankincense, Oregano, Lavender, Geranium, Fennel, Tea Tree** and **Basil** all help. By far the easiest remedy, that works like a charm. Simply get a large cabbage leaf, fold it into two, and place it in your bra cup. Replace every 2 – 3 hours. Cabbage leaves are cooling in nature and will help drain out the infection.

But here is a suggested recipe to massage into the breasts 2 or 3 times a day. Remember to wash thoroughly if still breastfeeding: **2 drops Geranium, 2 drops Fennel** and **2 drops Lavender** in 12 mls Almond carrier oil.
Other considerations – Diet, underwear, antiperspirant.

MENOPAUSE: Use in a diffuser or for massage in base oil. **Basil, Geranium, Ylang Ylang.**
Other considerations – Diet, Exercise, Vitamin Supplements.

MOUTH ULCERS: Mix 2 drops **Peppermint** oil, 2 drops **Thyme** oil, 2 drops **Lemon** oil, 2 drops **Tea tree** oil, 2 drops **Geranium** oil into 10 ml brandy and a glass of warm water. Mix thoroughly and swill around the mouth 2 or 3 times daily.

NAIL INFECTIONS: Combine 1 drop **Tea Tree,** I drop **Tagetes,** 1 drop **Oregano** with 5mls of carrier oil such as **Jojoba oil, Almond oil** or a base cream. Massage the blend into affected nails. Dab and soak a cotton ball or a cotton swab in the blend and apply it covered with a plaster for up to 5 hours. Repeat daily until the infection subsides and completely disappears.

OEDEMA: Make up 50mls lotion or oil with 10 drops of **Grapefruit**, 10 drops of **Lemon,** 5 drops of **Cypress**, 5 drops **Fennel,** and 5 drops of **Geranium** = 35 drops. Apply twice daily to affected areas. **Lemongrass, Chamomile German, Frankincense,** and **Juniper** also help.
Other considerations: Reduce salt and caffeine and drink lots of water and dandelion tea. Increase foods that contain magnesium.

PMS: Mix 5 drops **Clary Sage,** 5 drops **Marjoram** and 5 drops **Ginger** into 20 mls **Almond** or **Calendula** base oil. Massage into stomach and pelvic area. **Lemon, Rose** and

Geranium are also useful.

Other considerations: Diet, exercise, vitamin supplements, warmth.

PREGNANCY: The following oils should **NOT** be used during the pregnancy at all mainly because of their Ketone and Phenol content and although none have been proved to be harmful (except in large doses) it is unwise to use any of the following oils or any oils that you are not completely familiar with: **Angelica, Aniseed, Basil, Camphor, Cinnamon, Clove, Fennel, Hyssop, Lemongrass, Myrrh, Nutmeg, Oregano, Sage, Thyme, Tarragon, Pennyroyal, Wintergreen.**

Oils that should be **AVOIDED** in the first 6 months: **Juniper, Lavendin, Marjoram, Cajuput, Caraway, Clary Sage, Rosemary, Cypress, Myrrh, Niaouli, and Pine.**

The following oils **CAN BE SAFELY USED** during pregnancy (after the first 3 months): **Bergamot, Chamomiles, Frankincense, Grapefruit, Geranium, Lavender, Orange,** and **Ravensara.**

These oils can be used safely during the whole pregnancy: **Cedarwood, Neroli, Eucalyptus R, Ginger, Tea Tree, Lemon, Sandalwood, Mandarin, Rose Otto, Petigrain, Ylang Ylang.**

Essential oils do cross the placenta but have been filtered by the time they reach the foetus. The placenta is extremely selective and because they are natural molecules, the body knows how to deal with them.

Morning Sickness: 1 drop of **Peppermint** in a glass of honeyed water first thing in the morning.

General Nausea: Use a burner with a mixture of **Eucalyptus Ginger** and **Lavender**. A lovely smell, relaxing, uplifting and antiseptic. Also try **Sweet Orange** and **Petigrain.**

Stretch Marks (prevention): Mix 100 mls chosen carrier oil (**Almond, Grapeseed, Coconut**) with 7 drops of each. **Lavender, Mandarin** and **Frankincense** or **Neroli, Lavender** and **Chamomile.** Liberally apply from neck to knees daily.

Insomnia: Only use **Lavender** (angustifolia) 2 drops on a pillow at night. **Sandalwood** and **Ylang Ylang** in a vaporiser in the bedroom before retiring can help too.

Back Pain: Use any of the oils that are safe for pregnancy before 6 months. Use 5 drops of each **Rosemary** and **Lavender** in a warm bath, or the same mixed with 50 mls of carrier oil for massage after the first 6 months. Try **Roman Chamomile** and **Lavender** together too.

Mood Changes: There are many conflicting emotions during pregnancy that are both confusing and upsetting for the mother. Essential oils are marvellous to help lift spirits. 10 drops of **Clary Sage** oil on a tissue tucked into the bra can keep moods at bay and help the mother remain cheerful and alert. **Geranium, Rose Otto, Neroli, Chamomile** and

Jasmine are also good for balancing the emotions.

Preparation For Labour: Towards the end of pregnancy around the 8th month some of the previously forbidden oils are excellent. **Sage and Fennel** strengthens the womb. **Cypress and Rosemary** will ease aching limbs. During labour, make a treatment oil of **Rose Otto, Geranium and Clary Sage or Rosemary, Neroli and Frankincense** and use to massage the patient's back, arms, hands and legs. Both mixes are wonderful for the nervous system and facilitate easy breathing. The calming effect increases the oxygen supply to the blood and brain and helps the woman avoid hyperventilation. They are also antiseptic and disinfectant.

For a foot massage use **Chamomile, Sandalwood and Mandarin** in a dilution of carrier oil to relax during the waiting period. **Ginger** if nauseous.

Try 1 or 2 drops of **Neroli, Peppermint, Basil** mixed together in a diffuser or vaporiser.

POST NATAL CARE: Cracked Nipple Oil: Use only pure **Almond or Calendula** oil.

Healing the Perineum: 5 drops of **Cypress** and 5 drops of **Lavender** in the bath. Neroli is good too but best applied in a cream: 1-2 drops to 10mls cream.

To Promote Lactation: An ancient remedy for promoting lactation is to chew Fennel seeds and although it has not yet been established scientifically the use of the following oils can be tried **Fennel, Clary Sage, Lemongrass.** Use a mix of oils: 15 drops to 50 mls carrier oil and massage gently around the breasts into the armpit regions every day. Wash thoroughly before feeding the baby.

To Stop Lactation: 5 drops **Cypress,** 5 drops **Peppermint,** 5 drops **Lavender** with 50 mls carrier oil. Applied 3 or 4 times daily.

Haemorrhoids: 6 to 8 drops of **Cypress** in the bath.

Post Natal Depression: The following oils strengthen the nervous system and lift depression: **Bergamot, Neroli, Clary Sage, Grapefruit, Geranium and Rose.** Try a mixture of **Rose, Bergamot and Clary Sage or Geranium, Neroli** and **Grapefruit.** Mix together in a separate bottle and simply add a few drops of oil to a diffuser. Use the blend in the bath or mixed with a carrier oil for a massage.

Essential Oils to Use After a Miscarriage: Choose a single oil or blend mix – **Rose Otto, Frankincense, Geranium, Grapefruit and Chamomile.**

SINUS: Suggested recipe: **Tea Tree, Eucalyptus, Oregano, Cedarwood or Peppermint** in a diffuser. Try 5 drops in a diffuser or in hot water for sinus relief. Choose your more soothing oils for hot water inhalations usage, like in steam bowls, as hot oils could become quite irritating to the nasal passages used this way.

Other considerations – Diet, Chemicals, Congested tears.

SKIN PROBLEMS:

Acne: Mix 50mls **Aloe Vera Gel** with 10 drops of any of the following: **Bergamot, Frankincense, Lemon, Lemongrass, Chamomile, Juniper**, **Oregano, May Chang, Patchouli, Grapefruit** or **Peppermint**. Or add 10 drops of **Tea Tree**, 2 drops of **Rose** and 2 drops of **Lavender**. Apply 2 or 3 times daily.

A good combination is **Oregano**, **Rose** and **Lavender** with **Tea Tree. Oregano** oil contains carvacrol, an active compound with excellent antimicrobial properties that can help to kill acne-causing bacteria, dry out acne lesions, and reduce swelling and inflammation. It is especially beneficial against cystic acne; a severe type of acne that usually occurs in the teenage years, where pores become clogged leading to large pimples, chronic inflammation, and infection. **Tea Tree** is a more powerful as an antiseptic than carbolic acid or phenol (chemicals that are antibacterial, antiviral and antifungal). **Rose** essential oil though expensive has been used for centuries for any sort of skin condition. **Lavender** oil is so versatile that it can be used for almost any complaint. It is non-toxic and non-irritant.

Other considerations: Diet, stress, age.

Eczema Dry: Add 5 drops **Geranium** and 5 drops **Chamomile** to 12 mls of cream or good base oil.

Eczema Wet: Add 5 drops **Juniper Berry** and 5 drops **Lavender** to 12 mls of **Aloe Vera** or good base oil.

Other oils that help: **Bergamot, Hyssop, Patchouli, Neroli,** and **Rose**.

Other considerations: Stress, diet, life-style, sensitivities.

Psoriasis: Not easily helped, but as it is sometimes a stress related condition the relaxing oils help. **Bergamot, Chamomile, Geranium, Lavender, Peppermint, Benzoin, Patchouli, Sandalwood and Oregano** oil help to alleviate symptoms, and although there's no official published research on this, it may well be because these oils are natural anti-inflammatories. Aloe Vera applied to the skin up to three times a day helps reduce redness and scaling. Look for creams containing 0.5% aloe. Bathing with a handful of Oats, Dead Sea or Himalayan Salt in the bath can alleviate itching.

A suggested recipe: Add 2 drops **Bergamot,** 2 drops **Patchouli**, 2 drops of **Chamomile** or **Benzoin** to 12mls **Almond, Calendula** or **Hypericum** base oil. Apply daily.

Scars: For general scarring try the following: into 50 mls **Coconut oil** add 50 mls **Aloe Vera,** 10 drops **Lavender** and 10 drops of **Frankincense** and 10 drops of **Mandarin**. Add I capsule of Vit E and one Vit A. Whip together and apply daily. Other oils that help are **Thyme, Bergamot, Chamomile, Patchouli, Rose** and **Geranium.**

Sunburn: 10 mls **Aloe Vera Gel,** 5 mls **Hydrosol,** 2 drops **Lavender.**

SKIN CARE

Cleansing exfoliator: 2 teaspoons of oatmeal or mixed nuts finely ground in a food processor so that it resembles course sand. Add ½ teaspoon of cider vinegar and a pinch of salt plus 2 drops of your chosen oil. For oily skin try **Lemon, Lavender, Tea Tree, May Chang** or **Geranium**. For dry skin, **Clary Sage, Chamomile, Geranium** or **Patchouli** and add ½ teaspoon of Almond oil. Gently roll the mix over your face with your fingertips and then rinse thoroughly. This will remove dead layers of skin and help reduce clogged pores.

Body Lotion for dry and aging skin: This particular lotion is full of vitamins and is known to hydrate the skin well. 30 mls **Olive oil**, 30 mls **Coconut oil**, 2 tablespoons **Shea butter**, 2 tablespoons **Vitamin E**, 4 teaspoons of **beeswax.** Add 40 drops of your chosen oils. **Geranium, Mandarin, Orange, Chamomile**, **Lavender, Patchouli, Rose** and 20 drops of **Cinnamon** essential oil. Start by melting the base oils, beeswax and shea butter together by putting them in a glass or china bowl. Place in a saucepan with water and heat gently until melted. Refrigerate the mixture at least for an hour for solidification. Take it out and whip it till it's fluffy and add essential oils and vitamin E to the mix. Fill the lotion into a bottle and store in a cool place. Apply liberally after a bath or shower

Rich Moisturiser for dry skin: 1 teaspoon **Lecithin** (which is high in natural fatty acids and good for all skin types.) soaked overnight in 25 mls **Hydrosol**. 1 desert spoon of

Beeswax, 40 mls **Almond oil,** 5 mls **Vitamin E oil,** 5 mls **Evening Primrose** oil and 5 mls **Jojoba.** Melt the oils and wax together in a double boiler. Whip in the hydrosol with lecithin until the cream starts to cool. Add 20 drops of **Lavender** and 20 drops **Patchouli** and whip again. Sterilise some glass jars before placing the cream in them. Store in the fridge until use.

Note: Hydrosols are floral waters sometimes called Hydrolats. They are the by-products of essential oil distillation. They are available in a variety of aromas including rose, orange or jasmine. If you wish to make your own floral water you can add 100 mls of boiling water to a handful of fresh or dried Lavender, Melissa, Marigold, Mint or Rosemary. Leave to cool, strain and use straight away, as it will not keep well using this method.

Special Amaranth Cream for Hardworking Hands & Feet: 2 Tablespoons of **Beeswax**, 2 tablespoons of **Shea butter**, 2 Tablespoon of **Coconut** oil, 2 tablespoons of **Almond** oil, 1 teaspoon of **Amaranth** oil. Melt oils and beeswax together in a Bain Marie. Whip until the consistency of thick custard and then add your chosen essential oils. 12 drops **Geranium**, 12 drops of **May Chang** and 5 drops of either **Vanilla** or **Lavender.** Mix thoroughly and decant into sterilised jars.

Simple cream for face and body: 1 teaspoon of **Beeswax**, 1oz of solid **Coconut** or **Shea** butter, 20 mls **Jojoba** or **Almond** oil, 20 mls of **Hydrosol**, 10 to 15 drops of any of the skin oils. A few drops of isopropyl alcohol will extend the life of the cream, as it is an excellent preservative. Prepare as above.

Eye Gel: Mix together 30 mls **Aloe Vera**, 1 teaspoon of **Avocado oil** and ½ teaspoon **Honey**. Add 4 drops **Frankincense** oil. Whip together and place in sterilised jar.

Face wash: This is an unusual and effective face wash for spots and blemishes. 1 tablespoon **Coconut** oil, 2 tablespoons **Honey** (preferably raw)**,** 1 teaspoon **Apple Cider Vinegar,** 15-20 drops **Cinnamon** or **Geranium** essential oil**,** 2 capsules of live probiotics (if you have them).
Mix all the ingredients using a hand blender till it's a smooth paste. Your face wash is ready to use. Bottle it up and keep in a cool place. A small amount, the size of a pea, will cleanse the whole face and neck. Rub in for a minute and rinse thoroughly.

Facemask for all skin types: 1 desert spoon of **Fullers Earth** or finely ground **Oatmeal** mixed to a paste with a **Hydrosol** of your choice. Add 3 or 4 drops of essential oil. **Patchouli, Neroli, Lavender Bergamot, Geranium** or any of the citrus oils. If your skin is very dry add a small amount of Almond oil. Apply and leave for at least 15 minutes. Rinse off thoroughly.

Toner for dry skin: 100 mls **Hydrosol,** 25 mls of **Witch Hazel** (a natural astringent). Add 10 drops of any of the oils recommended for dry skin conditions. Shake really well before use and use a cotton wool pad to apply.

Toner for oily skin and blemished skin: 75 mls **Hydrosol** 50 mls of **Witch Hazel.** Add 10 drops of any of the oils recommended for oily and blemished skin conditions. Shake really well before use and use a cotton wool pad to apply.

STOMACH UPSET: There can be many causes of an upset stomach, such as indigestion, bacterial infection, excess acid, bloating and more. Toxins and bacteria can cause inflammation of the stomach lining, and the anti-inflammatory oils will help ease pain and aid in digestion by enhancing the release of bile and gastric juices.

Oregano oil has shown to be effective against several strains of bacteria such as e.coli and salmonella, the microbes notoriously responsible for causing food poisoning. **Tea Tree** inhibits most bacteria. **Peppermint** is anti-inflammatory and antiseptic. These three together can work wonders. For severe stomach upsets, add one drop of each to 10 mls olive oil. Mix well and drink quickly.

For the elderly or children use external application. Mix 2 drops of each of the oils into a cream or base oil and massage into the stomach 2 to 3 times daily.

SUNBURN: Mix 1 drops of **Peppermint,** 2 drops of **Chamomile** and 2 drops of **Lavender** into 8/10 mls of **Jojoba, Almond** or **Hypericum Base** oil or a pure lotion base. Other oils that help: **Orange, Geranium, Rose** and

Frankincense. Apply to affected area.

TEMPERATURE: Normal temperature is around 99° F or 37° C although this fluctuates during the day, during activity, relaxation and illness. Any oils described as Rubifacient will raise the body temperature such as **Black Pepper, Juniper, Marjoram, Thyme** and **Rosemary.** Oils that will lower body temperature are **Bergamot, Frankincense, Grapefruit, Lavender, Eucalyptus, Peppermint** and **Orange.** Add to a bath or a diffuser.

VARICOSE ULCERS: The following treatment has been found to be successful in the treatment of ulcers. In the bath, any of the following: **German Chamomile, Lavender, Geranium and Tea Tree.** Diluted with water to spray on affected area: **Eucalyptus, Geranium, Lavender and Rosemary.** Shake well before use. Mixed with carrier oil for dressings: **German Chamomile, Lavender, Geranium and Tea Tree.**

VARICOSE VEINS: Apply before rising in the morning the following mixture. Mix 100mls oil or lotion with 7 drops of each **Cypress, Lemon** and **Lavender,** 10 drops of each **Geranium** and **Cypress. Frankincense, Lemon, Rosemary, Patchouli** in the bath.
Other considerations: Diet, Exercise, Relaxation.

VERRUCAS: There are many types of warts. All are caused by the HPV virus, regardless of their location and name. But there are two main types: plantar and "regular" warts. Plantar warts are called verrucas and are one of the more common warts and, by definition, are only found on the feet while other varieties of warts are found elsewhere on the body. It's important to note that if you are dealing with genital, anal or warts on the larynx that you should seek medical attention. Those warts are a bit more precarious and need special care. There are quite a few oils that can fight off the wart virus including **Tea Tree, Clove, Lemon, Eucalyptus, Cedarwood, Lavender, or Cypress.** Treat warts by using a cotton bud and neat **Lavender** essential oil. Mix 12 drops of any of the above with a teaspoon of base oil and massage into warts three times daily. Others have found mixing 2 drops **Lemon,** with 10 drops of **Cider Vinegar,** which can be put onto a gauze dressing.

WOUNDS: Do not apply directly onto wounds but massaging around the area is best. A spritzer spray can also be

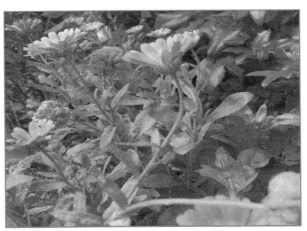

used on leg ulcers or open sores. Remember that essential oils and water do not combine, so shake vigorously before applying. Any of the following oils can be used, as they are all Antiseptic and Vulnerary: **Benzoin, Bergamot, Frankincense, Geranium, Neroli, Patchouli, Lemon, Rosemary, Tea Tree,** and **Lavender.** For small scratches

115

and cuts clean with **Tea Tree** on a piece of cotton wool and apply neat **Lavender** to promote healing.

Calendula oil will help heal the skin. (**Calendula** is shown on the previous page).

ABOUT THE AUTHOR

In her working years, Joy Burnett was a practising Aromatherpist, Reflexologist, and Holistic Healthcare Practitioner.

In 1990, she worked with AIDS patients for Cleveland Aids Suppport and wrote a clinical thesis on the immune system, some of which was published in Shirley Price's 'Aromatherapy for Health Professionals'.

In 1993, Joy opened her own school in North Yorkshire, 'The Rainbow Bridge School of Aromatherapy', accredited nationally by ISPA the Internation Society of Professional Aromatherapists and taught to a high level of expertise.

For over 11 years, Joy taught and practiced her art there and in other schools. Her students studied Aromatherapy for 14 month and were encouraged to extend their knowledge in other natural disciplines, some of which were offered at her school. They included Anatomy and Physiology, Reflexology, Indian Head Massage, Nutrition and the Chemistry of Essential Oils.

Many of her graduates became known in the North East as professional healthcare practitioners working alongside the NHS, supporting their work with children, cancer patients, in hospices, with pregnancy and the elderly, improving the relationship between modern and traditional medicine.

Now retired, Joy writes, directs amateur theatre, enjoys her pets and travelling.

Having lived in Oman, Brunei, Abu Dhabi and Spain, she now lives in Northamptonshire.

After joining a local writers group, Joy was inspired to start writing and produced her first novel 'On The Loose'. Others are planned and will be published soon. She has also written a short story collection 'All at Sea' about holidaying on a cruise ship. These books are available on Amazon.

Note from Joy Burnett:

Thank you for purchasing Healing with Essential Oils. I hope you have found it useful. I would be very grateful if you would leave a review on Amazon. Thank you.

If you have any questions about the contents of the book or would like to know more about my writing, I would love to hear from you.

My email address is joyburnettwriter@yahoo.co.uk

Printed in Poland
by Amazon Fulfillment
Poland Sp. z o.o., Wrocław